the Pro-Nurse Handbook

Designed for the nurse
who wants to ~~survive~~ *thrive* professionally

Melodie Chenevert lives and works in Gaithersburg, Maryland. She directs her own company, PRO-NURSE, that provides products and services designed to increase professional pride and productivity. In addition to the *Pro-Nurse Handbook*, she is the author of *STAT: Special Techniques in Assertiveness Training for Women in the Health Professions; Mosby's Tour Guide to Nursing School*, a survival guide for nursing students; and a coloring book called *I Might Be a Nurse* to introduce children to the many roles nurses play. Her latest book is a career planner titled *What Next Nurse?*

As a professional speaker she has conducted workshops throughout the United States as well as in Canada, England, and Australia, focusing on communication skills, management strategies, creativity, and innovation.

She received her diploma from Methodist-Kahler School of Nursing in Rochester, Minnesota; her bachelor's and master's degrees from the University of Washington-Seattle with a clinical specialty in psychiatric nursing; and an MA in Journalism from the University of Wisconsin-Madison. Before forming her own company, she worked as a staff nurse, play therapist/child mental health clinician, instructor in psychiatric nursing, and even set up an entire school of nursing from scratch.

THIRD EDITION

the Pro-Nurse Handbook

Designed for the nurse
who wants to ~~survive~~ professionally
thrive

MELODIE CHENEVERT

Illustrated

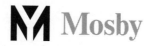

Mosby

St. Louis Baltimore Boston Carlsbad Chicago Naples New York Philadelphia Portland
London Madrid Mexico City Singapore Sydney Tokyo Toronto Wiesbaden

Mosby
Dedicated to Publishing Excellence

A Times Mirror
Company

Vice President and Publisher: Nancy L. Coon
Executive Editor: N. Darlene Como
Senior Developmental Editor: Laurie Sparks
Project Manager: Deborah L. Vogel
Production Editor: Jodi Willard
Manufacturing Manager: Theresa Fuchs

THIRD EDITION

Printed in the United States of America
Composition by Proof Positive/Farrowlyne Associates, Inc.
Lithography/color film by Proof Positive/Farrowlyne Associates, Inc.
Printing/binding by R. R. Donnelley & Sons Company

Mosby–Year Book, Inc.
11830 Westline Industrial Drive
St. Louis, Missouri 63146

Library of Congress Cataloging-in-Publication Data
Chenevert, Melodie, 1941–
    Pro-nurse handbook : designed for the nurse who wants to
survive/thrive professionally / Melodie Chenevert. —3rd ed.
      p. cm.
    Includes bibliographical references.
    ISBN 0–8151–1215–7
    1. Nurses—Job satisfaction. 2. Nursing—Psychological aspects.
I. Title.
    [DNLM: 1. Nursing. 2. Career Mobility—nurses' instruction.
3. Interprofessional Relations—nurses' instruction. WY 16 C518p
1997]
RT82.C49 1997
610.73'019—dc20
DNLM/DLC
for Library of Congress
                        96–24753
                        CIP

96 97 98 99 00 / 9 8 7 6 5 4 3 2 1

To
Gary, Eric, Ryan, Panzer, and Pandora

Third Time's a Charm

Whenever it's time for a new edition, Mosby asks me if I have any suggestions for the cover. Yeah. A plain, brown wrapper!

The *Pro-Nurse Handbook* has a "pssssst . . . pass it on" quality. It's been smuggled into hospitals and schools of nursing. It's a book that has been eagerly passed from hand-to-hand by what I like to call the "Nurses Underground Network"—a network that consists of real-world nurses working in the trenches and struggling to make sense of nursing's nonsense.

Nothing gives me more pleasure than to autograph a dog-earred copy and hear, "This book saved my sanity" or "Just when I thought I was going to have to leave nursing, a friend gave me this book."

The *Pro-Nurse Handbook* is often controversial. It provokes thought. Best of all, it incites action. It is designed to break through the victim mentality that stunts the growth of so many promising nurses.

Revising it's been tough. Changes in our industry and our society are coming so fast and furiously, it's impossible to know what nurses in the near future will find useful and relevant. It's not just that everything could change before I finish revising this book, everything could change before you finish *reading* this book!

In this edition you will find some facts, some truths, some trends, some rumors, some speculations, some suggestions. Take what you need and leave the rest.

As you grapple with the issues and incidents presented, keep in mind what Karl Menninger said about loyalty:

Loyalty means not that I agree with everything you say or that I believe you are always right. Loyalty means that I share a common ideal with you and that, regardless of minor differences, we fight for it, shoulder to shoulder, confident in one another's good faith, trust, constancy, and affection.

As nurses we share a common ideal: safe, sane, humane health care.

Hopefully, everyone who reads this book will become "pro-nurse." Each will be able to stand up and say, "I am a professional. I am an advocate for nurses and nursing." And each will look for ways to demonstrate, nurse-to-nurse, evidence of "good faith, trust, constancy, and affection."

Melodie Chenevert

Pssssst . . . pass it on!

Prologue

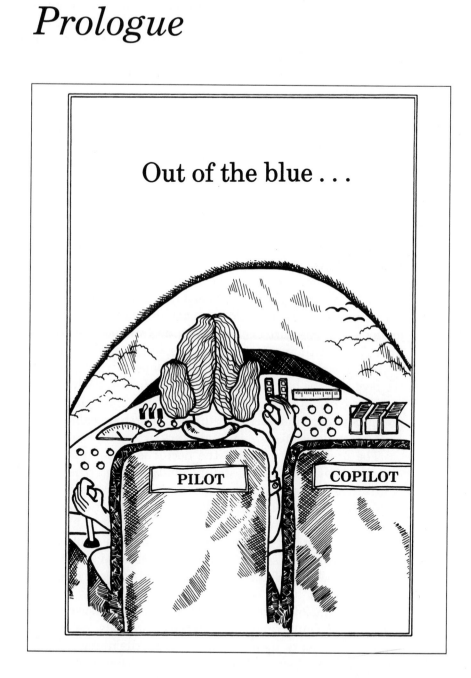

Being admitted to the hospital is much like boarding an airplane. The cost is sky high. Once on board you must relinquish control to the crew. You must trust their judgment, follow their schedules, and adhere to their rules. Whether passenger or patient, you pray for a safe landing at the desired destination.

Your contact on the plane is almost exclusively with the flight attendant. She greets you, seats you, comforts and feeds you. In the hospital the nurse performs similar functions. Perhaps that's why she is so easily mistaken for a "stewardess."

Pilots, like doctors, are essentially inaccessible. Occasionally their voices boom over the loudspeaker announcing the speed, altitude, weather conditions, and estimated time of arrival.

Over the years passengers have come to rely on the flight attendant for their comfort and on the pilot for their safety. In much the same fashion, patients have come to rely on the nurse for their comfort and on the doctor for their safety.

In an analogy between a hospital unit and an airplane, it is not surprising to find the doctor assuming he's the pilot. Whenever analogies of this sort are proposed, doctors assume the key position. They see themselves as captains, kings, or quarterbacks.

The hospital administrator also leaps to the conclusion that the doctor is the equivalent of the pilot. He sees doctors, like pilots, as necessary. He may see nurses, like flight attendants, as nice but not necessary. Nonessential nurses: interchangeable, disposable. Hospital policies often reflect this view.

The nurse also assumes the doctor is in the pilot's seat. She scurries about the cabin smiling and serving. When turbulence occurs, she goes forward to the cockpit. To her horror she finds it empty. She slides into the pilot's seat, not out of choice but out of necessity.

She is catapulted from flight attendant to pilot. Hearing the passengers ring for service, she is confused. Which is *real* nursing? Cabin or cockpit? She shuttles back and forth trying to do both jobs at once.

Her confusion is compounded by space-age doctors who beam aboard at irregular and unpredictable intervals. They materialize for a few moments, demand to know why the nurse is in the pilot's seat, and order her to return to the cabin where she belongs. The nurse complies.

Before long the plane goes into another tailspin, and once again she finds herself in the pilot's seat. She sits uneasily. She never wanted to steer. She just wanted to serve. Yet in real life the nurse is more analogous to the pilot than the doctor is.

Think about it. In this analogy the doctor cannot be the pilot for one simple reason. He is not on board. Actually, the doctor is more analogous to ground control. Essential but absent.

Nurses know getting in touch with ground control is difficult at best. The communication system is unreliable. Messages are garbled. Even when contact is established, nurses often get nothing but static. (As long as doctors and administrators insist on flying by remote control, they would be wise to upgrade the communication system and stop downgrading nurses.)

A veteran pilot quipped that flying is 95% boredom and 5% sheer terror. Fortunately for the pilot, his compensation is not based on 95% of the flying he does. His compensation is based on the 5% he hopes he doesn't have to do. He is compensated for those times when he must override automation and exercise all his training, skill, judgment, and experience to correct errors, minimize complications, and avert catastrophes.

Nursing, like flying, is 95% routine and predictable. Almost automatic. But nursing also has its 5% sheer terror. Unlike the pilot, unfortunately, a nurse is compensated based on the routine and predictable (cabin duties). She is not rewarded for her training, skill, judgment, or experience. She is not recognized for correcting errors, minimizing complications, and averting catastrophes (cockpit duties).

Imagine saying to a pilot, "Look, you and I both know that superb engineering has made flying almost automatic. Sure we need an expert's touch for takeoffs and landings, but in between you've got a lot of time on your hands. Once you're sure the plane is on course, go back into the cabin and serve refreshments. Make sure everyone's happy. But keep one eye on the instrument panel just in case something goes wrong."

Any pilot would tell you to take a flying leap. Pilots know how to provide service without being subservient. Nurses must learn to do the same. It's a matter of survival.

Science and technology have gifted us with gizmos, gadgets, and all sorts of mechanical miracles. Without the proper human connection, however, they are utterly worthless.

Reading meters, graphs, and gauges takes skill. Reading

patients takes even more skill. Nurses must be able to do both. We must monitor the machinery and mind the patients. We must be well versed in "high touch" as well as "high tech" care.

We must be able to detect a subtle slowing of activity, a grimace, an involuntary twitch, a faint odor, a slight variation in respiration. We must read between the lines. We must hear the unspoken word.

Many changes, most too minuscule for the unskilled eye or ear, signal the need for minor corrections. Failure to make those minor corrections can lead to major malfunctions. For airplane passengers the results range from discomfort to death. The same is true for hospital patients. It matters not whether the error is caused by inexperience, ignorance, or inattention. The result is the same.

Now, from out of the blue, come DRGs and other cost-containment policies forcing hospitals to carry full loads of complex patients from sickness to wellness in record time. Nurses fear the result will be roughly equivalent to having patients "deplane" at 1000 feet. The knowledge that we brought them down safely the first 34,000 feet is small consolation.

If our patients are to survive, nurses will have to stay in the cockpit, where we can see clearly and effect safe landings. Cabin-bound nurses can't set the course or change directions. They just get taken for a ride.

It's precisely because we have spent more time in the cabin than in the cockpit that our profession is in a crash-and-burn configuration. Unless we assume command, we may not survive. Unless we learn to command well, we will not thrive.

The *Pro-Nurse Handbook* is designed to help you pilot your own craft. Don't keep flying by the seat of your pants. Learn to fly first class.

Jettison your flight-attendant complex, strap yourself into the pilot's seat, and prepare for turbulence. There may be some rough weather ahead, but remember, you can't reach great heights without climbing through the clouds.

◆   ◆   ◆

Contents

Chapter 1

Pros and Cons

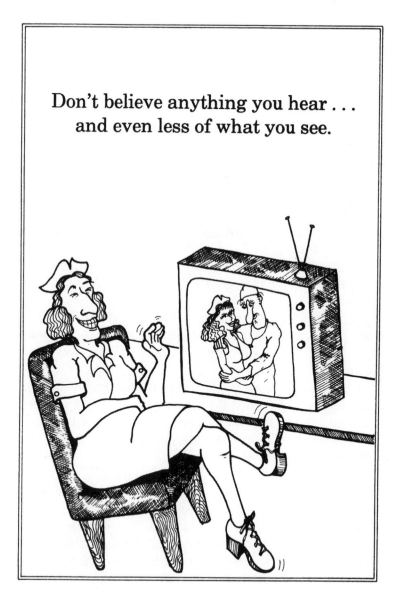

Fool me once, shame on you.
Fool me twice, shame on me.

How do a couple of sharp professionals like you and I get conned so easily and so often? Is it because we're too gullible, too naive, too nice, too trusting, too unsure of our own judgment or worth? Yes!

♦ We've been conned into believing that nurses are a nicety, not a necessity, and that we could be replaced in an instant.

Employers have held this threat over our heads for years. Yet even when nurses were in critically short supply, we didn't call their bluff. Why? Because we're too flea-brained.

Let me explain. I have it on good authority that when you first put fleas in a jar, they vigorously jump up and down banging their little heads on the lid. It hurts! Those determined little buggers quickly learn to adjust the height of their jumps. They continue to leap about, coming within a hair's breadth of the lid.

After a couple of days you can remove the lid, and the fleas won't jump out of the jar. They continue to jump just short of where the lid was.

We nurses have a lot in common with those fleas. After years of low ceilings and painful encounters, we have learned to jump only so high. Even when the lid is removed, we won't jump out of the jar.

Sometimes I think the lid hasn't been removed at all, we've just been conned into thinking it has. On my more pessimistic days I suspect the tin lid has merely been replaced by one of transparent plastic. Today we can see new heights, but we can't reach them.

From all the talk about liberation, equality, and professionalism, you'd think we could easily escape the jar. But when we jump higher, we still bump our heads. We still hurt.

Actually, very little has changed. For example, women still account for 99% of all secretaries and 1% of all plumbers. The gap between men's and women's wages has decreased. A woman now makes 70 cents to their dollar. Unfortunately, this is not because women's salaries are increasing. It is because men's salaries are eroding.

Women are still the ones with dishpan hands. And nurses are still "just nurses" and not the full partners in the health care system that we have longed to be.

> ◆ We've been conned into believing that we are the descendants of prostitutes and Florence Nightingale died of syphilis.

As nurses we are woefully ignorant of our history and what little we know, or think we know, serves to embarrass us. It makes it difficult to take pride in nursing.

I am not a history buff but it rankles me to hear nurses belittle "Flo." If we had more nurses like her we could take over the world. She was intelligent, well-educated, articulate, assertive, politically astute, goal-driven, tenacious, persistent, respected, and successful.

In a Canadian bestseller *The "I" of the Hurricane: Creating Corporate Energy,** author Art McNeil discusses vision and values, challenge and response, fostering individual commitment, action plans, and achievement by design. He gives six leader profiles to illustrate his points: Winston Churchill, Thomas J. Watson, Sr., Napoleon, Mahatma Gandhi, Martin Luther King, Jr.—and Florence Nightingale.

Sometimes it seems that those outside of nursing appreciate her abilities and accomplishments more than those of us inside the profession.

> ◆ We've been conned into believing that politics is a nasty business that is better left in the hands of men.

According to the National Women's Political Caucus, women are "tragically underrepresented politically." While women make up more than half of the population, they comprise only 8% of the Senate and only 11% of the House of Representatives. Those small numbers help explain why we continue to have such ineffective policies on education, child care, and health.

The lack of women in political office was never more glaringly apparent than during the Clarence Thomas confirmation hearings. Lynn Yeakel won an upset in the Pennsylvania Senate Primary by

---

*McNeil, Art: *The "I" of the hurricane: Creating corporate energy,* Toronto, 1988, Stoddart.

running tapes of the incumbent, Arlen Specter, grilling Anita Hill and then asking voters, "Does this make you as angry as it makes me?" It did. The voters gave her the victory.

While nurses have advised politicians about health care issues for years and have held local and state offices, no nurse served in Congress until 1993 when Eddie Bernice Johnson of Texas took her seat in the U.S. House of Representatives.

A number of nurses with impressive credentials and track records are poised to run. Like Johnson they are committed to making health care available to all. They are tackling tough issues concerning the aged, children, victims of violence, substance abuse (including the epidemic of drug babies), apathy about breast cancer, crime, jobs, education, and affordable housing. Substantive issues.

If nurses want choices, if we want to make decisions and establish policy, we must not only be politically astute, we must be politically *active*. Maybe you and I will never be candidates ourselves, but we can support the nurses who are. We can stuff envelopes, telephone, ring doorbells, shake hands, and shuttle people to the polls—anything to help get out the vote.

And we can donate money. Remember, there are over two million of us. Think what would happen if every nurse donated ten dollars!

One nurse told me she felt a bit guilty writing out a check to a political candidate without first discussing it with her husband. When she mentioned it at dinner, he said he had made a contribution to a candidate for another office that day as well. Her check was for $100. His was for $1,000! End of guilt. She thought about it and then wrote out a check for another $900.

Would you be surprised to learn that former Senate Majority Leader Bob Dole's chief of staff is a nurse? I was. And, it was working on the substantive issue of welfare reform that landed her in hot water and in the headlines. The headline in the *Washington Post,* August 11, 1995, read:

> "Sheila Burke, on the Wrong Side of the Right. Dole's Embattled Top Aide Is a Nurse. Good Thing."

Evidently, she was under attack from ultraconservative, right-wing Republican groups who were demanding Dole get rid of her. They resented her position and her power. They called her a "spawn of militant feminism" and worried that she was manipulating him toward becoming—horror of horrors—a "moderate."

A former senator who worked closely with her, David Duren-berger of Minnesota, says, "She's found a way, which very few peo-ple who ever worked for Bob have found, to be a counsel to him and get the job done, and be somebody he actually can trust. Sheila *is* Bob Dole. If anybody has any criticism, they can direct it at him, because she is not an independent agent."

In answer to her critics, Sheila said, "There's never been a time when he (Dole) doesn't control what goes on. Staff are staff in every sense of the word. I don't think anyone who works for him is ever confused."

Dole "stoutly champions his aide," but he's not the only one. *Democratic* Senator Robert Byrd of West Virginia eloquently defended her on the Senate floor. It seems she is respected by both Republicans and Democrats. Supporters from every camp describe her as incredibly bright with an awesome memory for details, unquestionably competent, rock solid, and extremely knowledgeable on legislative procedure and policy issues. They also say she is "tough-minded" and "has a Margaret Thatcher–like intensity."

This petite, blonde, fortysomething mother of three young chil-dren obtained her nursing degree from the University of San Fran-cisco. After working in Berkeley, she moved to New York to become program director of the National Student Nurses Association.

Even though she was a "congenital Democrat," she came to Washington in 1977 to work on Dole's personal staff tracking health issues. She stayed on and in 1986 was named chief of staff. Because of her enormous respect for Dole, she eventually changed her party registration to Republican.

In his excellent article, staff writer Lloyd Grove says, ". . . in the Senate she most often resembles a triage nurse, giving short shrift to the politically dead and dying in order to attend to the politically recoverable."

It's now 1996 and Dole is running for President. We may be hearing more about Sheila Burke. Stay tuned. And, let's hope the next article on her isn't relegated to the "Style" section of the paper.

If you're ready to get more involved politically, you might want to participate in the Nurse in Washington Internship. The four-day experience is guaranteed to demystify the legislative process. Con-tact the National Federation of Specialty Nursing Organizations in Pitman, New Jersey (609-256-2333).

♦ We've been conned into believing that money is not the most powerful substance on this planet.

When I hear women denying their need for monetary reward, I am reminded of cognitive dissonance theory. The theory says that when your beliefs and your experience are at odds, you feel pain. Brain pain. Your mind seeks resolution.

If you can't change your experience, you alter your beliefs so there is less disparity. If you find you don't have much money, you simply tell yourself that you don't need much money. Since women know they can't earn nearly as much as men, they deny money's importance. Then they expend great effort searching for another means to validate their worth in a society that sees them as "worthless."

Seeking to avoid pain, we lower our expectations. The lower your expectations, the less likely you are to be disappointed. Unfortunately, if you expect to be poor, you will be. If you expect to be mistreated, you will be. You'll be poor and mistreated, but you won't be disappointed because you got what you expected.

To thrive, you have to have high expectations. If you set your sights on mole hills, you will never conquer mountains. *Moral: think mountains.*

♦ We've been conned into believing it's more important to be liked than respected.

A man who works with his hands is a laborer.
A man who works with his hands and his head is a craftsman.
A man who works with his hands, head, and heart is an artist.
And a woman who works with her hands and her heart is a
   nurse.

Give St. Francis credit for the first three lines. The last line is to no one's credit. Unfortunately, we've been conned into believing that nurses don't need heads, just good hands and big hearts.

While screening applicants for admission to nursing school, I was surprised and appalled by the low quality of many applicants. They couldn't read, "right," add, or subtract. I hesitated to even suggest they seek employment as beauticians or manicurists because I didn't think most of them should be allowed to handle sharp objects. Yet they were told by friends, relatives, and *high school counselors* that they would make good nurses.

♦ We've been conned into believing nursing is a duty, not a career.

Recalling a bit of her own ancient history, an older nurse wrote,

I was called in to scrub around midnight. At the time we were paid three dollars a call whether it was for 1 hour or all night. When I grumbled, the surgeon chastised me, saying I should be "happy to serve."

Naturally he was making several hundred dollars to my measly three. I told him that when I was paid as well as he was, I would be "happy to serve." Happy? I'd be hysterically happy!

♦ We've been conned into believing that hard work, like virtue, is its own reward.

I wish I would have been more assertive when I recently got a new job. As my boss (a man, of course) and I were discussing my salary, it actually came down to being slightly less than my present salary. I made a statement to him, "That's OK. I don't want this job only for the money," and I accepted the job with an actual cut in pay!! Ouch! A promotion?

When a new hospice was being organized, the community sponsoring it assumed they could get a master's-prepared nurse to voluntarily direct it. They were told by nurse advisors that was utterly ridiculous. After all, there was an acute shortage of nurses, and those with advanced degrees were particularly scarce. Evidently their prayers were answered because they found one.

For a full year that nurse directed the hospice on a part-time basis under the supervision of a chaplain. Finally, she rebelled. Her "part-time" involvement consistently topped 40 hours a week. The salaried chaplain's "supervision" consisted of a once-a-week "How ya doin'?"

The last straw came at a banquet when she found herself handing out awards to volunteers. Her anger bubbled to the surface as she admitted to herself that she had indeed been taken. For all her work she was not even getting a token award.

The volunteers never dreamed that such a highly professional person was going without a salary. The salaried people—chaplains and counselors—who worked alongside her never offered any appreciation or praise for her efforts.

After months of subservient service, she demanded the directorship be removed from the chaplain's supervision. The director would only be accountable to the board. She also demanded the position be made full-time and carry a respectable salary.

Today the hospice is a highly successful operation. She continued to run it for 4 years but she directed it as a paid professional, not as a volunteer.

Would she do it again? Probably. The need was so great and the patients' gratitude so rewarding, almost any nurse would have trouble resisting. I would. I'll bet you would too.

Unfortunately, our profession will not thrive as long as we are more duty bound than career bound. We will not be taken seriously by other professions until we lay claim to the reward and recognition that should accompany our hard work.

♦ We've been conned into believing the doctor is always right.

Hospital rules

1. The doctor is always right.
2. If the doctor is wrong, see rule 1.

Every so often I see a bumper sticker that reads QUESTION AUTHORITY. Unfortunately, nurses have been so conditioned to believe that the doctor is always right that even under circumstances in which a doctor's behavior is outrageously inappropriate, most nurses will conform instead of confront.

The following was submitted by a nurse as an example of a time when she *wished* she had been more assertive:

> A doctor who works part-time in our clinic wanted to turn off the lights to do a pelvic exam on a woman because he said he could focus in on the vaginal canal with his head lamp.
>
> I felt it was inappropriate but did so anyway. I felt uncomfortable during the entire exam because I could not see what was going on. I had to assume the doctor was acting appropriately. I hoped the patient would not be uncomfortable or scream "rape!"
>
> When I tried to talk to the doctor later and tell him how I felt, he exploded.

This nurse failed to challenge the doctor on the spot because she questioned her own authority. She had self-doubts about her own knowledge and experience.

Any doubts this nurse had should have vanished when the doctor "exploded" as she tried to discuss the situation with him. He knew he was out of line.

Faced with a similar situation, a nurse has several choices. She can refuse to turn out the lights, she can strap on a head lamp of her own to monitor the patient and the doctor ("Gotcha!"), or she can enthusiastically suggest that they write up his unusual practice methods for publication since no other doctor seems to share his views.

> One doctor rants and raves about "poor nursing care" on our unit in front of patients, visitors, and nurses, then storms off. I am left standing speechless by this unexpected attack and angry that I didn't "do something."

We have been conned into accepting abuse because, like battered wives, we think we have done something to provoke it. We think it must be our fault. Horsefeathers! The man's a jerk. Being a physician merely makes him a "professional" jerk.

It's not a matter of the nurse being too sensitive or the doctor being too insensitive. There's a lot more at stake here than rudeness or hurt feelings.

The doctor has cast aspersions on the quality of care being offered by those nurses, on that unit, and in that hospital. Being a physician, his words carry a lot of weight. The damage he is doing is impossible to calculate, but it is considerable. Situations like this start visions of malpractice suits dancing in my head.

Can you for one moment imagine the tables turned? Can you imagine a nurse deriding a physician in front of patients, visitors, and other doctors?

"Geez, what a quack! I wouldn't let you operate on my dog! Where'd you buy your diploma anyway? Don't you ever botch things up like this again, or I'll have you thrown off my unit!"

You can bet those would be the last words ever uttered by that nurse. At least, her last words as an employed nurse.

> A patient (demanding, manipulative, wealthy) complained to her doctor that the nurses had been telling her what she was and was not to do! (This is a cardiac rehabilitation unit where we monitor a patient's response to gradually increasing activity.)
>
> The doctor, upon hearing her complaint, stormed into the station demanding that "one of the girls" explain what happened. Meek little me who always wants to smooth things out agreed to go into the patient's room with him to talk this out.
>
> The doctor and I returned to the room. His statement to the patient was, "This one will apologize for all of the nurses. Now don't

pay any attention to the nurses. They don't know what they're talking about. You just listen to me."

I was so upset I couldn't speak. Later, when I tried to talk to the physician about what had happened, he replied, "Well, that's how you have to handle a woman like that."

This doctor has been conned into believing that women—nurses and patients—have to be "handled."

♦ We've been conned into believing there is a health care team.

The dictionary defines teamwork as "work done by several associates with each doing a part but all subordinating personal prominence to the efficiency of the whole."

Nurses can easily set aside personal prominence. We have so little, it's not much of a sacrifice. Doctors, on the other hand, enjoy a great deal of personal prominence. To set theirs aside is a major sacrifice.

Every day, health care professionals attired in various uniforms traipse out onto the playing field. Since we don't practice together, we are never sure of just what the game plan is. We never know what our teammates are going to do next.

Some hog the ball. Others insist on running toward opposing goals. No one seems to know the score. Watching doctors and nurses play, you'd hardly know we were on the same side.

It was brought to the attention of the staff nurses that the doctors felt the nurses weren't treating them as professionals and were being unprofessional in their conduct. I suggested that a meeting be held with a panel of doctors and a panel of nurses to air our problems. The idea was put down by the medical staff and dropped.

What was the purpose of this skirmish? Certainly it served no useful purpose. Quite the contrary.

Here is a skirmish in which doctors and nurses worked together to score a touchdown:

We were having problems with both doctors and nurses when it came to accurately recording intakes and outputs. The day shift blamed the night shift for errors. The night shift blamed the evening shift. Talking about the importance of I & Os did little or no good.

The doctors were irate. They griped constantly. They wrote on the doctor's orders in big, bold, black letters: **DO I & O AND RECORD.** They "bad mouthed" the nurses in their weekly medical meetings. The problem continued.

Our solution? We created a task force composed of three doctors and three nurses (one from each unit in our department) to meet, discuss the problem, and propose solutions.

Group communication was open and heated. Each person aired his or her feelings. Immediately there was change for the better. After 6 months, the situation had improved so dramatically that the medical staff highly commended the nurses for their effort.

The task force has remained operational. Problem-solving has been an ongoing process. The group deals with any problem, large or small. There are no more temper tantrums. The doctors and nurses have become real partners in patient care, and everyone is much happier.

Finding a multidisciplinary team that is alive, well, and fully functioning is a rare but exhilarating experience. Such teams are founded on intense mutual respect. Often all members are on a first-name basis. Information flows freely. Decision-making is shared. Members take turns being "captain" based on patient needs at the time.

Peter Drucker, who writes extensively on management topics, likens the development of a new organization to a symphony orchestra. That's a wonderful analogy for the health care team. In a symphony orchestra every group plays different instruments but they all have to come together voluntarily, they all have to play in harmony, and they all have to know the score. The only difficulty I was having with the analogy was figuring out who would be conductor.

I finally decided it would have to be the patient, who would be standing up front, clutching his open-air gown closed, and waving the baton. Because one of the things we keep forgetting is that the patient is the most important member of the multidisciplinary health care team.

When there is discord, the patient suffers. If every nurse, doctor, dietitian, housekeeper, social worker, and lab technician would focus on the patient, we could make beautiful music together.

♦ We've been conned into believing that we are not only responsible for everyone's health and well-being, we are responsible for their happiness too.

♦ We've been conned into believing that health care is a right. Furthermore, we've been conned into believing it is our responsibility to provide that care cheaply, abundantly, and eternally.

At a conference on geriatric nursing, a clinician told of a dilemma posed by a cantankerous 85-year-old woman. The woman had a history of COPD, right CVA with left hemiparesis, multiple MIs with CHF, and renal failure. As if this weren't enough, she was also an insulin-dependent diabetic with a seizure disorder.

As each medical crisis arose, she was rushed from the nursing home to the hospital. There they patched her up. As soon as she stabilized, they shuttled her back to the nursing home.

Once back at the nursing home, she indulged in all the former vices, which precipitated the need for emergency care again . . . and soon! She smoked incessantly, sometimes polishing off three packs a day. She ate only what she liked. She had an insatiable craving for salty foods and sweets. She was also overly fond of alcohol.

The health care team began to tire of building her up only to have her tear herself down again. She had them trapped in a vicious circle. They knew they couldn't win, but their code of ethics made it impossible for them to walk away from the game.

She died leaving over $150,000 in unpaid hospital bills. Everyone agreed the money was less important than the huge amount of professional time, talent, and energy she had consumed.

Money, time, energy—once spent they cannot be recaptured to invest in another person. Accepting the fact that these precious resources are *limited* is the first step in allocating them wisely. One way to conserve is to stop trying to save people who don't want to be saved.

Out of necessity the pendulum is swinging. Although once viewed as a right, health is being seen as a responsibility. Each individual's responsibility.

♦ We've been conned into believing . . .

Nice nurses don't _____

Good nurses do _____

(Fill in the blanks yourself.)

Next time you're with a group of nurses, ask them to define a good nurse by finishing this sentence in 25 words or less: "A good nurse is a person who . . . . " There are two conditions. First, everything said must be positive, and second, there can be no tasks in the definition.

You will quickly realize how much nurses define themselves by the number of tasks they are able to accomplish in any given time period. Leaving any task or chore unfinished seems to negate the value of those completed. A nurse driving home at the end of a shift is not congratulating herself on all she got done; she is kicking herself for all the things she left undone. She is barely conscious of all the patients and families she helped. Instead she is focused on the one patient or family she couldn't help.

♦ We've been conned into believing that it is more important to correct our weaknesses than to capitalize on our strengths. That's why we are always apologizing and homogenizing.

When I was being interviewed for a job in mental health, I was asked about my "tendency to be aggressive or assertive." They asked me to promise "not to make waves."

♦ We've been conned into believing it doesn't matter who gets the credit as long as *we* know we've done a good job.

I worked in public health in an "unorganized county," which means we do not have a county health department.

We had a food poisoning outbreak and did all the follow-up that was needed. We wrote the reports and did a "super job."

The local town health officer called us in and asked for a copy of all our reports. Then he promptly told us he would make the report to the state capitol for us because we did not have a physician on our staff and therefore were not "qualified" to answer any questions the state epidemiologist might ask.

Until we stand up and take credit for our good works, no one will know how much nurses actually do or are capable of doing.

In an effort to contain costs, a CEO suggested to the vice president of nursing that she reduce her professional nursing staff. He claimed their mix was "too rich" and should be diluted with cheaper, nonprofessional help.

Before discussing it further the nurse executive insisted that the CEO and the board of directors follow a nurse for a half-day to see what professional nurses did on a moment-to-moment basis.

You can imagine how carefully she chose her nurses for this assignment. They were all Level 4 on the clinical ladder. She instructed them not to take on an extra heavy load or do anything out of the ordinary. All she wanted them to do when they had the VIPs in tow was to "think aloud."

When the tour was over the CEO and the board members were so impressed, they withdrew their request. To a person they were amazed by all the split-second decision making and critical problem-solving nurses did. They came away with a new appreciation of what quality care really is. They decided there were better ways to reduce costs than by reducing their professional nursing staff.

All nurses need to be encouraged to "think aloud." We need to speak up so people know we are not hired hands—we are hired for our brains.

Slogans like "Nursing: The Heart of Health Care" always irritated me because it takes so much more than heart to be a good nurse. To deal with my frustration I eventually produced a poster showing a pediatric nurse reading *The Wizard of Oz* to two children with the caption "Nursing: Courage, Heart, Brains."

A man called to order that poster for his wife for Nurse's Day. She had admired it and he wanted to surprise her. He said he liked it too, except for the "brains" part. When asked if he didn't think his wife was smart, he stammered, "Well, yes, but . . ."

Nurses? Brains? Nurses are not often credited with smarts.

During workshops I have been asking nurses to share examples of courage, heart, and/or brains in action. Here are a couple of my favorites.

I can't speak the language of the critical care nurse who was sharing this example but it was one of those situations in which the patient was rapidly going from bad to worse. The room was packed with nurses, doctors, respiratory therapists, and technicians. Everyone's adrenalin was pumping. Nothing they tried was working. High drama.

They were contemplating heroic measures that would not really prolong life but would prolong death. At that moment the head nurse walked into the room and said quietly, "Ladies and gentlemen, we have viable patients across the hall who are dying."

Treatment was suspended. Everyone paused for a moment of silence for the patient they were losing. Then they dispersed and went about caring for the patients who did have a chance to survive. Tough call.

Courage, heart, brains.

Another example came from an OB nurse. A very pregnant young woman who had been in a long and losing battle with cancer was admitted to their unit. Her only goal now was to live long enough to deliver her baby. They cared for her for a couple of weeks and then it was decided to airlift her to a big metropolitan hospital.

It was there her baby was born, but it did not survive.

The doctor called the head nurse at the small community hospital to tell her that the patient was returning and had requested to be placed on the OB unit. He said, "You don't have to take her. It's not even an appropriate placement. There's no longer a baby involved."

The head nurse said, "Hold just a moment." Then she quickly polled all her nurses. To a person they said, "If she wants us, we want her." So the dying woman came back to their unit.

Stop and think about why nurses choose OB. They love to see life begin. We have other nurses who are expert at helping patients at the end of life. Oncology nurses. Hospice nurses. This had to be a difficult time for all of them.

The young woman kept asking questions. The nurses kept reassuring her. Yes, she had done everything right. Yes, she had done everything humanly possible to have a live baby. It just wasn't to be. Yet no amount of reassurance seemed enough. The questions kept coming.

Then one of the OB nurses said, "Well, maybe she just needs to see babies." They bundled up the fragile young woman, put her on a cart, and took her to the newborn nursery. As they watched her interact with the babies, they suddenly realized she had never been allowed to grieve for the baby she had lost. She had been actively dying so long herself, and everyone was so focused on her, that when her baby died no one seemed to notice.

Those OB nurses helped her write down her thoughts. Then they conducted a memorial service for her baby in the hospital chapel. A few days later she slipped into a coma and died on the OB unit.

Courage, heart, brains.

After you grab a Kleenex, I'll end this little section on a lighter note. A head nurse in the ER shared this wonderful example. This was the problem: a doctor would do a procedure and leave a mess. When the nurse cleaned up, she might be stuck by a needle or blade hidden in the debris. In this day and age, if you are stuck by a "sharp," it truly can be life-threatening.

To the head nurse the situation was intolerable. She decided to sponsor a month-long contest she would call "Zero Tolerance for Sharps." She created a poster-sized grid with each doctor's name listed down the left side and the days of the month, 1–31, across the top. Then she got smiley-face stickers and frowny-face stickers.

After a procedure was done, she would check the room. If the doctor cleaned up and left no sharps, he got a smiley face. If he left a sharp, he got a frowny face.

At first the doctors laughed it off. Did she really think they would fall for anything so hokey? She told them to do whatever they wanted. She just kept putting up the stickers.

It turns out doctors don't like to see frowny-face stickers behind their names. They started cleaning up. Pretty soon it got to the point where a doctor would corner the head nurse and demand to know why he got a frowny face. After all, he had cleaned his room. Then the head nurse would show him the sharp that had been found and he'd apologize, insisting it wouldn't happen again.

When the contest began, there were predominantly frowny faces. In a few days the mix began to change. There were more and more smiley faces. After a couple of weeks there were predominantly smiley faces. Toward the end of the month, day after day, there were *all* smiley faces. They had achieved "Zero Tolerance for Sharps." The contest was over. The head nurse took the poster down.

The very next day, a doctor came up to her saying, "I cleaned my room." He was looking all around for the poster. He wanted his smiley-face sticker!

Courage, heart, brains—and humor.

One of the things I learned while getting a master's degree in journalism is that health-related articles are the most frequently read articles in any magazine or newspaper. Yet how often have you seen a byline with "RN" attached? Few nurses ever write for the popular press.

A more alarming commentary is that journalists rarely, if ever, seek out nurses as sources of information on health care. That's the conclusion of a fascinating study by the Women, Press & Public Policy Project in Cambridge, Massachusetts.

After analyzing 423 articles on health care that appeared in the *New York Times,* the *Washington Post,* and the *Los Angeles Times* during the first quarter of 1990, researchers reported that of 908 sources quoted, nurses were at the bottom of the ranked list with only ten quotes. That's about 1 percent, which means almost 99 percent of the information in those articles came from non-nurses (doctors, government officials, business people, medical organizations, educators, patients, etc.). Nurses were even out-ranked by a nondescript category labeled "workers"!

The authors found it especially disturbing that nurses were virtually ignored even in health care issues in which nursing plays a critical role. For example, a nurse was the main source of information for only *one* of the ninety articles on AIDS, and no nurses appeared as source authority for *any* of the articles covering "disease prevention . . . access to care, drug addiction, chronic illness, maternal-child health, right to die, geriatrics, and informed consent—areas in which nurses are also central and responsible for major program innovation."*

Two days before I read this article, a nurse executive shared her disappointment at being unable to convince the human resources department to provide funding assistance for a staff nurse who wanted to pursue a degree in journalism. They just didn't get the connection. They thought it was an inappropriate course of study for a nurse. I sent her the article, hoping that even if it were too late to help the last nurse, she would be better able to help the next nurse.

In a spring 1992 editorial, Donna Diers of Sigma Theta Tau's journal *Image* cites the above study and then offers examples from her local newspaper and a popular radio call-in show in which nurses were slighted. She tells about hearing an internist on the talk show attempt to field a question from a woman who had received a nonsensical diagnosis from a doctor about a painful knee. As he struggled to find a tactful way to encourage her to get a second opinion, Diers says, "I thought, too briefly, about calling in to get him off the hook to say something like *I am a nurse* and I know this diagnosis is meaningless and your caller should defi-

---

*Buresh, Bernice; Gordon, Suzanne; and Bell, Nica: Who counts in news coverage of health care? *Nursing Outlook* 39:204–208, Sept–Oct 1991.

nitely see someone else. . . . It was an occasion to make nursing visible, and I hate to confess I went on stirring my chili and let it pass."

How many of us have gone on stirring the chili and letting things like that pass?

Diers also says it is not that "nurses are not knowledgeable or that we aren't talking. The problem is, people aren't asking."

Typical, isn't it? Polite, passive nurses standing in the shadows waiting to be asked. And, even if they are asked, being afraid to speak up, terrified they might be wrong. Once again doubting our own knowledge, skills, and experiences.

Nurses need to be more visible and more vocal. The premier issue of *Revolution—The Journal of Nursing Empowerment,* published by Laura Gasparis Vonfrolio, debuted in spring 1992. The cover featured a group of nurses with no mouths.

Maybe we need to be more mouthy.

Laura was also the driving force behind the nurses' march on Washington, D.C., on March 31, 1994. Police estimated the crowd at about 35,000. Nurses came from every part of the United States to call attention to hospital downsizing and restructuring that could result in unsafe patient care.

They were alarmed by the growing numbers of RNs being replaced by unskilled workers. They came to sound the alarm to politicians and to the public.

It must have been an impressive sight. Unfortunately, I missed it. By the time I learned of the march, I had a speaking engagement locked in across the country. My husband promised to tape the evening news.

I arrived home at midnight and the first thing I did was plug in the tape. Nuts! Gary had taped his favorite news, the MacNeil-Lehrer Hour on PBS, instead of our local Washington-area news. They flashed a few seconds of the nurses' march as the lead-in to their segment on staffing concerns at a California hospital.

Saturday morning I jumped out of bed and grabbed the *Washington Post*. There was nothing about the march. "Ahhh," I thought, "it's such a big story they're saving it for Sunday." The 10-pound Sunday edition arrived. Nothing. "Ahhh," I thought, "they're saving it for Tuesday and their health magazine insert." Tuesday came. Nothing.

Evidently, they're still saving the story. For readers of the *Washington Post,* the march never happened. It's perplexing. A handful of peeved poodle groomers could protest and get more coverage.

If you missed the march too, you can get a video from ANA. Perhaps they should have sent a copy to the *Washington Post.*

It's not enough to speak up. We have to make sure we are heard.

Leaders of this historic event realized that one march wouldn't be enough to change anything. They exhorted nurses to return to their home states and continue speaking out personally, professionally, and politically.

Anonymous nurses will never be considered essential. Nursing will not thrive until our contributions are acknowledged by the more respected professions, by the politically powerful who shape policy, and by the public at large.

Nurses can also be great con artists. Here's a wonderful example to share:

> We had just moved into a brand-new hospital building, and nothing seemed to be going right. The tube system failed, the diet carts were late, and the medications disappeared in the transport system.
>
> The nurses were overwhelmed. Patient census was high. Overtime was mounting. The doctors were irritable. Morale was in the pits.
>
> As head nurse, I was the target for disgruntled nurses, irate doctors, and unhappy patients. At the end of a particularly grueling day, a young surgeon approached. He proceeded to chew me up and spit me out.
>
> At first I was devastated. Then I was furious. Snatching a piece of paper from my desk, I printed "S–Doctor" in large letters at the top. I wrote the young surgeon's name on it and posted it on our bulletin board. In professional jargon, it was going to be my "excreta list."
>
> My staff nurses began to chuckle. One of the more artistic ones incorporated the "S" in a colorful Superman shield. Each day we added a physician's name to the list. There were so many who deserved the honor that choosing just one was difficult—but fun!
>
> The nurses went about doing their chores feeling very smug and smiling a lot. Morale went up 100 percent.
>
> As the days passed, I became a little concerned about our game. The doctors had obviously noticed the list. Some made a point of coming into the station to read it. At last one doctor cornered me and

asked about it. "Oh," I chirped, "that's our SUPER DOCTOR LIST." He asked me how to get his name on the list, and I told him the nurses voted at the end of each day.

From that day on doctors actually began competing with one another for the privilege of being on the list. They smiled, answered questions politely, asked if there was anything they could do to help. They engaged nurses in consultations, invited them along when they had something interesting to do, shared information from articles they had just read, and offered to teach in-service sessions.

Overnight, the list did become the SUPER DOCTOR LIST. And our doctors really became super.

Chapter 2

Promises, Promises....
and Other Propaganda

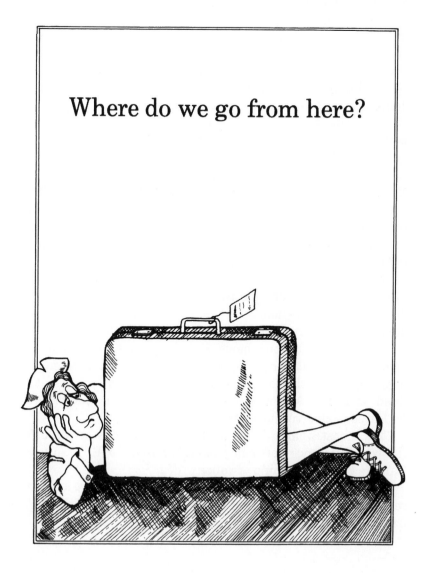

Where do we go from here?

Whither thou goest, I will go.
Wither thou lodgest, I will lodge.
Thy people shall be my people
And thy god, my god.

Oh, my god, we're moving again.

Some nurses are frustrated because they can't stay in one community long enough to establish a career. Others are frustrated because they are unable to leave their community to pursue a career. Women who find themselves in such a quandary have been referred to as "tied stayers" and "tied movers." As a woman who is definitely "tied" to a man, I have experienced both.

When my husband and I were married back in 1966, we were both in graduate school. Since he was an aspiring physicist, I knew the places he would be able to work were limited. We both thought it fortunate that I was a nurse and, therefore, *portable.* Nurses can get work anytime, anywhere. Promises, promises . . .

With each move Gary's career advanced: a better position, a better salary, and better fringe benefits. As the "portable partner," I trailed along happily. I managed to find or create jobs that suited my fancy.

As our sons were born, I fitted my "career" around our family life. I was more interested in flexible schedules than fringe benefits. I never questioned the salary offered. Opportunities for advancement were never even discussed.

It wasn't until our move a dozen years later that I really resented the whither-thou-goest clause in our marriage. I found myself exiled to the southeastern corner of Washington state. Sidelined. Derailed. Although there were "jobs" available, there were no "career" opportunities here for me.

Like most women I was well into my thirties before I grasped the real difference between jobs and careers. Jobs keep you busy. Careers build something of value.

After the last move, I began to recount my professional travels, reviewing my former jobs. Some were fun, some fascinating, some frustrating. All culminated in nothing.

While Gary was rewarded with each move, I was penalized. My

salary, vacation time, pension fund, level of responsibility, and place on the totem pole were reduced to ground zero. In each new community I had to start from scratch. I had to *prove* myself over and over again.

When I arrived in the never-green part of the Evergreen State, something snapped. I just didn't want to start all over again. Besides, we were only going to be here for 2 years. That was the plan. Unfortunately, we were there 9 long years.

Sometimes I feel like a helium balloon tied to an anchor. My husband provides a lot of security and stability. My problem is that I don't carry enough weight to budge him. When I shared this feeling with a friend, she suggested I just get a longer string. Now you know why I am so high strung.

When my husband and I entered our respective professions, our salaries were nearly equal. In our early years we used to talk about my finding the next job and his taking time off for other things. Soon that possibility became highly implausible. It would have been economically devastating for our family to try to live on my earnings.

Sadly, I've learned that jobs for nurses are plentiful but nursing careers are few and far between. "Go into nursing," I was counseled. "It's a good profession to fall back on." I guess they thought I would keep my nursing diploma in a box on the wall labeled IN CASE OF EMERGENCY, BREAK GLASS.

Education for a woman is often considered more like an insurance policy than preparation for a serious career. Our first duty is to be wives and mothers. If something should happen to our husbands (heaven forbid!), we would have a respectable means of making a living.

It's comforting to know I have a profession to fall back on. There are millions of "fallen" women out there who don't have any sort of marketable job skills to back them up. Millions who believed those promises of perpetual care so completely that they never learned how to take care of themselves.

Even though statistics show almost every woman will be forced to go it alone at some point in her life, we refuse to believe it. We fail to prepare ourselves emotionally, intellectually, politically, or financially.

Statistically speaking, you have almost a 50 percent chance of being divorced. Yet you have only a slim chance of being awarded alimony and, even if you are awarded child support, the odds on collecting it are disappointing (Census Bureau survey, 1988). Of the women who were supposed to receive child support, one fourth received the full amount, one half received partial payment, and one fourth received nothing at all. In 1990 the average child-support payment was only $44 per week.

A 1994 federal law mandated that employers could withhold child support payments from wages. It is similar to the way the IRS withholds taxes throughout the year. Perhaps this will help pull our nation's children out of poverty. Promises, promises . . . let's wait and see. Deadbeat dads are still making headlines.

Statistically speaking, you also have a *90 percent* chance of being widowed. So even if you are as lucky as I was to find a high-fidelity husband who promises you undying love, you can scratch the "undying" part. Try as we will, we just can't keep the little buggers alive.

Women still outlive men by an average of over 7 years. The average age of widowhood is 56. By age 65 half of all women are widowed. The Older Women's League (OWL) reports that only two of every ten women receive any pension based on their own or their husbands' earnings. If you don't want to wind up rummaging through trash cans for your next meal, you'd better plan ahead.

For instance, if you want to decrease or eliminate widowhood, you should marry a man 8 or 10 years your junior. Women in their twenties find that advice obscene, in their thirties laughable, in their forties conceivable, in their fifties preferable, and their sixties necessary.

Women who give up everything for love and men who give up everything for work eventually learn to their dismay that they based their lives on false promises. To thrive, a life must be built equally on both love and work.

Women have been told that entering the work place shoulder-to-shoulder with men will take years off their lives. Threat? Sounds more like a promise to me. If it ever comes down to a choice between quantity and quality of life, I'd prefer to go for quality. I'd rather lop 10 years off my life than spend them alone, poor, cold, sick, or hungry. Besides, there is no evidence to support that at all.

The best explanation of longevity I ever heard was a correlation between longevity and height. Short people live longer than tall people. That would explain why women as a group outlive men as a group. Because women as a group are shorter than men as a group. Also think about this—you go to the nursing home to see the "little, old people." There are no big old people!

Originally I thought my marginal salaries and minimal advancement opportunities were correlated with my disconnected work history. On closer examination I discovered that staying in one community and working for one institution would have made no difference. (It wasn't Gary's fault after all!)

As a woman and a nurse, I would have reached the peak of my earning potential within 5 to 7 years. Then, as "cost-of-living" raises failed to keep pace with the actual cost of living, my buying power would have steadily eroded.

So you see, I haven't lost much by being portable. I am just paying the heavy financial penalties this planet imposes on female occupants.

One spring I was unexpectedly offered an excellent position in a city I love. The salary was very respectable—for a nurse. Unfortunately, it was less than half my husband's salary. The "impractical" nurse in me longed to take the position. The "practical" nurse in me knew better.

I had just spent a year and a half setting up a school of nursing 300 miles from my home. The opportunity had been so unique that although I found it difficult to accept the position, I found it impossible to decline.

Gary backed me to the hilt. For the first time since our marriage I lived alone while Gary and the boys managed by themselves. Whenever possible I made a mad dash for home. Then our sons (Eric, 15 and Ryan, 11) elected to spend the school year with me. It was Gary's turn to live alone. It was his turn to make the long drive to be with his family.

Our phone bills were astronomical. After 18 months our tires and patience were wearing thin. Although our marriage was as strong as ever, we found long-distance parenting extremely difficult. It was with a strange mixture of grief and relief that I polished off the project and hired my replacement.

What an adventure! Would I do it again? Yes. Or so I thought until the phone rang and I was offered a wonderfully attractive position *only* 200 miles from home. That's when I realized I had not fully recovered. This time I declined. I had other promises to keep.

Women have been criticized for their high turnover rates, yet when consideration is given to the types of jobs that foster high turnover—low-paying, dead-end jobs with little opportunity for

advancement, marginal economic rewards, and minimal respect—
the turnover rate is the same for men and women.

It *appears* that women have higher turnover rates because we
have nearly cornered the market on crummy jobs—75% of all
women are employed in the service sector. And we're so cheap!
Take a man and a woman in the same crummy job. Give them
a *1 percent* increase in salary, and she is three times less likely
to quit than the man. Women continue to take jobs that no
self-respecting man would touch. That's because women are not
self-respecting.

We work hopefully ever after. Fairy tales taught us that a miserable life was mandatory if we wanted to marry a prince. They
promised us that no matter how poor, tired, hungry, overworked, or
underloved a woman was, Prince Charming was only a kiss away.

If you look closely at yourself, you might see a trace of Little
Red Riding Hood, Mother Hubbard, Sleeping Beauty, Cinderella,
Snow White, or other fairy tale characters.

Take Little Red Riding Hood. Are you the kind of nurse who gets
in trouble because you fail to follow directions or take foolish short-
cuts? Are you so nearsighted that you can't see danger (or opportunity) looming right before your eyes? Are you fair game for wolves?

Perhaps you're more like Mother Hubbard. Maybe you're the
kind of nurse who not only gives till it hurts, you give till it's gone.
You look after everyone's needs but your own. You're uncomfort-
able when people offer you compliments, assistance, advice, goods,
or services. Even when your cupboard is bare, you go through the
motions of giving even though it is just an empty gesture.

If you find the men you work for or live with come up short,
you have a lot in common with Snow White. Helping little people
is fine, but you don't want to work for one or marry one. Snow
White is cheerful, hard-working, and industrious but also naive,
compliant, and too trusting of the wrong people.

Sleeping Beauty closes her eyes to anything unpleasant or
strenuous. She dreams of a cottage, adoring husband, and
adorable children.

Rudely awakened by divorce, death, or the natural displace-
ment that occurs as children mature and move away, a Sleeping
Beauty often finds herself in dire straights—economically and
emotionally. She dozed off when she should have been paying
attention to insurance, investments, pension plans, personal development, and marketable job skills.

Like Sleeping Beauty, many nurses are dreamers. That's one of the reasons why our profession has not matured. In many ways nursing is for the young. First, it is strenuous: physically, emotionally, and intellectually. Second, the long hours and irregular schedule make it more suited to one who is personally unencumbered. Third, it requires exorbitant amounts of idealism and optimism. Fourth, often the advancement opportunities can only satisfy naive or immature professionals.

Many nurses prefer to keep their eyes closed, but some of us are quite alert. We are waking to find nurses cannot always get a job anytime, anywhere. Seeing that promise broken for the first time in the early 1980s and again in the early 1990s made many nurses feel betrayed. We were childish to believe nursing was a forever profession.

We were foolish to think unused knowledge and skills wouldn't decay. We were foolish to think women who walked (or ran) away from nursing years ago could step back in as if nothing has changed. We now realize that no one can fall back on nursing. You have to run to keep up.

Finally we're waking up, and we're growing up. After years of being politically unconscious, all Sleeping Beauties are showing signs of arousal. Until 1980, women had always lagged so far behind men in voting numbers that pollsters never bothered to include us in their surveys. By 1990 women were voting in greater numbers than men.

Gearing up for the 1996 elections, both Republicans and Democrats are worrying about how to attract women without alienating men. A GOP poll showed men believe government is "part of the problem" and women believe government is "part of the solution." The Republicans want a leaner government and they're afraid women will translate that as "leaner and meaner." Women already favor the Democrats, 38% to 29%.

"Women's Vote '96" is an alliance of 110 women's organizations ranging from the American Association of University Women to the YWCA. Their goal is to "make the women's vote the deciding vote in 1996." Emily's List (the name stands for Early Money Is Like Yeast) is planning to spend $10 million to help mobilize Democratic, pro-choice women voters. The National Organization for Women (NOW) will also be out in full force in a "Fight the Right" campaign.

Yes, we're awake, and we don't like what we see. We are just catching on to what politicians mean when they say, "Women and children first." They mean to throw us over the side of the economic lifeboat right along with the elderly and the infirm. Instead of closing our eyes and waiting for those same men to rescue us, we are voting in record numbers. From now on you can bet women will be polled.

There is another beauty in the Fairy Tale Hall of Fame: Beauty and the Beast. In this scenario men are beasts, and women are duty bound to save them.

When I was a student nurse on clinical rotation in Chicago, a psychologist speaking to our class said, "Nurses marry weak, dependent men." I was flabbergasted. By the time I got to the dorm, I was furious. How dare she say something like that!

As I grew calmer I began thinking about the kind of men I was attracted to—*losers*. There is something in me that responds deeply to need in others. I am drawn to people with handicaps, terminal illnesses, and quick but neurotic minds. I am a rescuer. Most nurses are rescuers.

The outspoken director of an alcoholic treatment center was discussing the types of people who make the best counselors. When nurses were mentioned, she blurted out, "Nurses? They're the worst! They always want to kiss everything and make it better."

Nurses work at salvaging human wreckage. Unfortunately, too many of us take our work home with us. We've been brainwashed to believe the love of a good woman can cure anything. We've been duped into believing that it is not only our duty to care for those less fortunate or able than ourselves, it is our duty to marry them! No wonder so few of us live happily ever after.

Once upon a time if you finished all your household chores, you got to go to the ball. If today's Cinderella gets all her household chores done, she gets to go to a job. Women account for almost 46% of the U.S. workforce.

Cinderella had her glass slipper; today's woman has her glass ceiling. In March 1995 the Glass Ceiling Commission, a bipartisan government panel, released findings of its 3-year study, which concluded that women still hadn't broken through barriers that keep them out of top management. Finding that 97% of senior managers at Fortune 1000 corporations are white males and only 5% of top managers at Fortune 2000 companies are women, the commission concluded the ceiling was "unshattered." Perhaps the most interesting finding was that the overwhelming majority of the CEOs they interviewed thought the problem had been solved!

Women are still waiting in the ashes hoping for a fairy god-mother to come along. We still believe it is magic, not money, that will transform our lives.

In her classic book, *The Cinderella Complex,** Colette Dowling talks about women's yearning for dependence. She feels the chief force holding women down is their deep-seated wish to be taken care of by others.

Two of the phrases in her book that particularly stuck with me are "collapse of ambition" and "dwindling into a wife." They are so descriptive of what happens to me and many other nurses.

For example, a group of highly credentialed coronary care nurses were complaining about being abused. They were exhausted from working double shifts, carrying heavy patient loads, and being forced to forego days off and cancel vacations.

Seeing their plight, a nurse administrator advised them to do what physicians had done long ago. She suggested they form a corporation and then sell their services back to the institution under their own terms. Immediately she witnessed what could only be described as a depressing "collapse of ambition" as every one of them "dwindled" into a nurse right before her eyes.

Those coronary care nurses could not see the opportunity presented by incorporating. They only saw the risk and danger. The thought terrified them.

Watching their courage and confidence evaporate, the nurse administrator felt very sad. Her hopes for nursing's eventual autonomy also dwindled. If highly educated, experienced, and talented nurses fled from autonomy, she doubted the rest of us garden-variety nurses could be expected to strive for it.

Fairy-tale women can be excused for being "Grimm." They're ancient history. Let's update our make-believe world a bit.

I love watching old movies on TV, but many of the lines uttered by my favorite leading men make me cringe. Lines like "Women and dogs—the more you beat them, the better they are" and "There are two kinds of women: mothers and the other kind."

Career women are not portrayed kindly, and no matter how successful they are, as soon as the male lead whistles, they drop everything and retire to the suburbs. When a classy woman is

---

*Dowling, Colette: *The Cinderella complex: women's hidden fear of independence,* New York, 1981, Summit Books.

being courted by two men, she invariably chooses the poorer, weaker one rather than the richer, stronger, more successful one. That's romance? That's stupid!

Every day we see John Candy dumpling–type men stroll off into the sunset with statuesque blondes. Just once I would like to see a plump, bespectacled woman (with a great personality) walk off with a Mel Gibson look-alike. But that will never happen. Why? Because nobody would believe it.

In vintage movies and television series, men used to have all the action, fun, and adventure. Today men still have all the action, fun, and adventure.

It begins in early childhood. Even in children's picture books, male characters have most of the action, fun, and adventure. A review of male and female characters in children's picture books published between 1976–1987* found that male characters far outnumbered female characters, were given the majority of central character roles, and were depicted in a wide variety of roles. Females were relegated to very limited, highly stereotypical roles such as teachers, old maids, housewives, and princesses.

Saturday-morning cartoons and toy advertisements continue to reinforce conventional sex-role definitions. Consider the Teenage Mutant Ninja Turtles. Even among nonhuman characters, males have all the action, fun, and adventure!

According to a 1994 University of Dayton study, male characters continue to dominate cartoons. They were portrayed as more active and adventuresome, while female characters were more compassionate and confined to domestic roles. Only 13 percent of the female characters had jobs, and male characters were never shown as caregivers. The researchers expressed concern that girls, at a tender young age, may already think their career choices are very limited.

A 1973 study of the portrayal of men and women in high school chemistry texts showed the books were "pervasively gender-biased, favoring men." To see if things had improved, the study was replicated in 1990. Of the seven best-selling chemistry texts, one had changed dramatically to become gender fair. The other six

---

*McDonald, Scott M.: Sex bias in the representation of male and female characters in children's picture books, *Journal of Genetic Psychology,* 150(4): 389–401, 1988.

were still biased, and in two cases had actually increased the proportion of illustrations favoring men.*

And we were promised things were changing.

No wonder preschool boys were upset when asked, "If you were a girl, what would you like to be when you grow up?" They couldn't think of anything worse than being a girl. "Yuck!" When preschool girls were asked, "If you were a boy, what would you like to be when you grow up?", they responded quickly and positively with dozens of different answers.

Women fare poorly on television. How do nurses fare? The made-for-television nurse had her prime time in the 1960s. An hour-long dramatic series, *The Nurses,* aired on CBS from 1962 to 1965. The series conveyed a highly positive image of the nursing profession, allowing nurses to be both compassionate and assertive, caring and intelligent, warm and decisive. The series also explored every facet and variety of nursing practice.

In the 1970s more nurses popped up on television shows than ever before. Unfortunately, they were more decorative than useful. They interacted with doctors instead of patients.

In the 1980s nurses were primarily "extras" and rarely main characters. They were still mostly decorative. They often served as the butt of practical jokes. They were also used as sponges to absorb verbal barrages from irate doctors. After all, someone had to listen to those self-righteous tirades writers love to pen for the script's doctor.

Then came *Nightingales,* a series that would more appropriately have been titled *Bimbos and Bozos Do Nursing.* Protests from nurses and nursing organizations managed to get the program removed. *China Beach* was a bright spot portraying nurses in the Vietnam War.

In the 1990s a situation comedy called *Nurses* debuted. My unofficial poll showed most nurses hoped for a quick demise. All of us wish we could have a program about nurses with writing and character development comparable to *L.A. Law.* Those lawyers may have had their personal problems but they were incredibly competent in their professional roles.

All scriptwriters would have to do is interview nurses and ask

---

*Bazler, Judith A., and Simonis, Doris A.: Are women out of the picture? *The Science Teacher,* 24–26, Dec. 1990.

them to describe one of their most unforgettable patients. They'd soon have more comedy, drama, action, and adventure than they could ever dream up. Truth is stranger than fiction.

Years ago I remember reading a first-person account in one of the nursing journals. I thought it would make a fantastic script. As I recall, a young man was bicycling in Florida when he was struck by a car. He sustained massive brain damage and had not a shred of identification on him. There was no way to notify his family and, in spite of publicity, no one came forward to claim him.

As he began to recover, all he could say was "1-2-1-2." The doctors and nurses tried to decipher what he meant. At first they thought perhaps 1 meant yes and 2 meant no. But that wasn't it. Then they thought it might be like when you raised your hand in school for permission to go to the bathroom and the teacher asked, "Number 1 or Number 2?" But that didn't pan out. They tested other theories and finally the doctors gave up. They said it was just gibberish. But you know how nurses are. We get something stuck in our craw and we can't let go of it.

One day a nurse came on duty and said, "What if it's an area code? What if he's trying to say '1-212'? That would be New York."

They brought the young man a phone and he punched in 1-212- and the rest of the number. That's how they found his family.

I'd say that's award-winning drama. Wouldn't you?

When NBC's blockbuster hit *ER* was launched in Fall 1994, it looked like nurses were going to be relegated to the handmaiden role once again. But the "nurses" quickly evolved from taking orders to giving orders and telling the doctors to "sign them." Nurses moved from the background to the foreground. In fact, one of the nurses became a lead character.

The changes came about because real health professionals who watched *ER* told the show's writers and producers early on that they were way off the mark. Today real nurses not only give technical advice, they often appear on the screen. Evidently some star-struck nurses are using their vacation time to try their hands at acting. According to Ellen Crawford, who plays a nurse (Lydia Wright), "Real nurses work in the trauma scenes. Usually if you see nurses working around the patient, but they don't talk, they're real nurses."

Chapter 3

Procreation

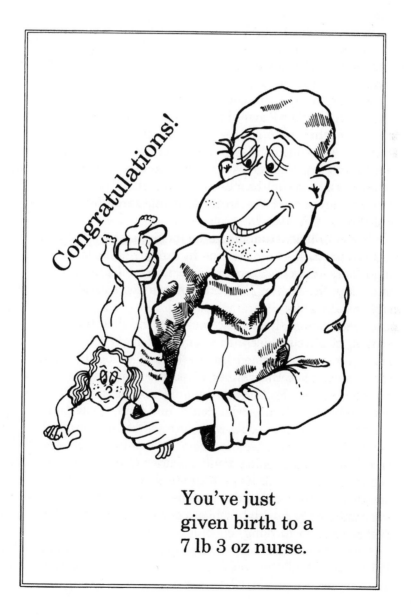

ARE nurses born or made?

Whether by birthing or by manufacturing, it takes 2 to 5 years of hard labor to bring forth a new registered nurse. The creation process requires one basic raw material: people. Finding people willing to undertake the study of nursing may be increasingly difficult.

First, the birthrate has declined. There are simply fewer young people approaching that critical first-career decision. All trades and professions are having to compete more vigorously for their share of the young.

Second, women are continuing to move into career fields previously dominated by men. Instead of choosing between being a secretary, teacher, or nurse, women are choosing to study computer science, accounting, law, and medicine. They are becoming mechanics, coal miners, truck drivers, and construction workers. Although the actual number adopting such "nonfeminine" careers remains miniscule, the trend is being carefully observed, highly publicized, and, ideally, encouraged.

Third, college students value money, status, and prestige. They are not particularly interested in the "joy of learning or the meaningfulness of work," according to annual freshman surveys conducted by the Higher Education Research Institute at the University of California.

These trends helped account for the fact that enrollment in schools of nursing declined every year from 1978 to 1987. Nurse educators were alarmed by the lack of students and even more concerned about the caliber of people applying for admission to nursing school. People who should not be permitted to handle sharp objects! People who could not read, write, add, subtract, multiply, or divide! People with zero science background!

High school counselors seemed to think anyone with a nice smile who liked people should consider a career in nursing. That's one reason I wrote *Mosby's Tour Guide to Nursing School*, which is basically a survival guide. The first few chapters have been used very effectively by high school counselors to help their students decide whether nursing school is a realistic choice.

One hospital not only invites high school students to a "Nurse Pal Career Day," they also invite their counselors. The counselors are very enthusiastic. They say it increased their awareness of things like job availability, practice areas, salary, educational levels, financial aid, and scholarships. They also said they were counseling a greater number of students to consider a nursing career.

Whole communities have teamed up to attract good students. In Indianapolis they have NURSING 2000, which services eight counties in Indiana. They sponsor "A Day in the Life of a Nurse," and in 1995 this event gave 500 high school students the opportunity to "shadow" a nurse. They work with counselors to make sure students in the program are taking appropriate science and math courses and are seriously interested in nursing. Over 200 nurse volunteers visit schools and other groups to talk about career opportunities.

What are you doing in your hospital, in your community, to recruit future nurses? In fact, what are *you* doing?

In 1990 Florida State University conducted a survey of high school students. Those students thought nursing was a low-status occupation and that nurses had difficulty finding jobs. Most said that nursing's benefits don't measure up to the time and money it takes to enter the profession.

Where did these students get their information? From watching nurses on television (30%) and from knowing and observing nurses (60%). It makes you realize the impact fictitious and real nurses have on recruiting the future generation. We may not be able to do much about nurses in the media, but we can certainly monitor our own behavior.

Because most nurses still *feel* overworked, unappreciated, and underpaid, this is the message we communicate. We scare off potential nurses. A niece or a neighbor expresses an interest in nursing school, and instead of encouraging them, we give them horror stories.

Every nurse needs to become an active recruiter. If you won't do it for altruistic reasons, do it for perfectly selfish ones. First, who do you want taking care of you and your family? Think about it. You are not only a health care provider, you are a consumer.

The other reason you need to recruit is because you are aging. The average age of the nurse now is 43 and increasing. Congress will soon rule that no registered nurse can retire unless she finds someone to replace her. So get busy!

Because there are not enough young people to go around, attention is being focused on people in their thirties and forties who are contemplating a midlife career change. Many men, disillusioned with their present jobs, are looking for more satisfying career alternatives. Many women, whose family responsibilities have decreased or whose financial obligations have increased, are looking at entering or reentering the job market.

The bulk of these people are not as naive as they were at age 18. They cannot afford the altruism of youth. They are asking serious questions about salaries, working conditions, fringe benefits, and opportunities for advancement. Can nursing attract and hold their interest?

The answer is a resounding "Yes!" In fact, the average age of today's nursing student is 29.

Many of the career-changers choosing nursing are doing so for one very important reason: job security. They have been out in the cold, cruel world and they know how tough it can be to find and hold a job.

By the early 1990s salaries in nursing had risen so dramatically and the national economy had deteriorated so drastically that people began clamoring for admission to nursing schools. People with brains and dexterity lined up at schoolhouse doors only to be turned away. Why? Because budget cutbacks meant there were not enough faculty to accommodate them. The "Labor Letter" column in the May 19, 1992, *Wall Street Journal* described this problem in Texas, Kansas, Colorado, Oklahoma, New Jersey, and California.

Just about the time we tooled up and got ready to accommodate the increased demand, the economy took another turn for the worse. This time it hit the health care field almost as hard as it hit other industries. Nursing salaries stagnated and job opportunities declined.

One thing we learned from the last go-round is that when nursing loses its primary appeal of job security, the grade point average (GPA) of students applying for admission to nursing school drops. Experts who track these trends say it's happening again.

Another disturbing trend is that the number of students entering bachelor's degree programs in nursing dropped for the first time in 6 years in fall 1995. According to the American Association of Colleges of Nursing, enrollment is down nearly 3%. The good news is enrollments in master's degree programs are continuing to rise because of increased demand for nurses with advanced skills.

My advice? If you want job security, you need either 6 weeks or 6 years of education. Certified Nursing Aides (CNAs) and Nurse Practitioners (NPs) are in great demand. For everyone in between it's a tough market.

In recruiting nursing students we have gone from famine to feast to famine. We must step up our efforts to make nursing an attractive career choice again.

The problems nurses encounter are a microcosm of the problems women encounter. Our profession is still 97% female. Facing the truth about life as a nurse may be as painful as facing the truth about life as a woman. Painful but necessary for survival.

While attending meetings of the American Association for the Advancement of Science, I happened upon a session concerning women and birth order. The speaker reported polls showing 80% of American couples, given a choice, would elect to have a male child first. She was concerned because there is evidence that firstborn children are likely to have higher IQs, better verbal skills, and a tendency to be high achievers.

As I listened, I began thinking about the field day science fiction writers could have with this piece of information. Imagine a future in which there are no firstborn females. Certainly technology enabling us to select the sex of our unborn children is imminent. Perhaps it is already available. . . .

My momentary daydream was interrupted when the speaker turned to the large, predominantly female audience and asked all the firstborn people in the room to raise their hands. A gasp went up as fully 95% of us, myself included, raised our hands. She simply nodded and said, "It happens every time."

As the session concluded, she left us with a haunting question: "Why don't women want to reproduce themselves?" That fascinating and frightening question still surfaces frequently in my mind.

Eventually her question coupled with the escalating nurse shortage triggered another question in my mind: "Do nurses want to reproduce themselves?"

While conducting workshops across the United States and Canada, I began looking for the answer. I asked hundreds of nurses to write their responses to the following:

"Your daughter (son) is about to graduate from high school. Give her (him) three convincing reasons why she (he) should consider becoming a nurse."

1. _____

2. _____

3. _____

Take a moment to fill in your own responses.

If you have difficulty coming up with three convincing reasons why *any* young person should consider a career in nursing, especially one as important as your own son or daughter, you are not alone.

After gathering the responses, I usually ask workshop participants how difficult it was to come up with three reasons. When given a scale from one to ten with ten being the most difficult, someone once chirped, "an eleven!"

> "I can't—I told both of my daughters not to go into nursing."
>
> "Encourage my son or daughter to go into nursing? *Never!*"
>
> "I really don't think I could give her three good reasons to become a nurse—in fact, I don't think I could give her *one!*"

One respondent wrote, "I spent 3 years convincing my daughter that there were other career fields offering her more respect, more pay, more personal rewards, and less physical exhaustion."

Another listed three convincing reasons *not* to consider nursing:

1. Society still thinks nurses are the brainless handmaidens of the world.
2. Nursing Education programs are worse than marine boot camp.
3. It is impossible to support a family on a nurse's salary.

With friends like these nursing doesn't need any enemies. The time has come to take a good look at ourselves and our colleagues. Are we walking advertisements for the nursing profession, or are we walking warnings discouraging people from considering nursing as a career?

Take your own poll. Ask the nurses on your unit, in your hospital, or at your nurses' association meeting to write down three convincing reasons for entering the nursing profession. You will easily identify nurses who are burned up, burned out, or still brimming with enthusiasm. Their responses make an excellent springboard for discussions of what's right and what's wrong with our profession. We urgently need to right the wrongs, so nursing can remain a viable career choice.

What's right with nursing? Even today, with our relatively tight job market, the *number one* reason given to encourage a son or daughter to consider a career in nursing is: "You can almost always get a job." In fact, "You can get a job anywhere in the world." Nursing is the most portable, packable credential you could have.

Have you been reading the advertisements for flying nurses? Sometimes I wish I were coming out of school unencumbered and could jet off and take one of those glamorous assignments. I thought it was too late for me until I met a nurse who is retiring in a year. She is reading those ads. That's what she is going to do. It is not too late for any of us.

Nursing is challenging. It taxes you to the limits. It is physically, intellectually, and emotionally demanding. Nurses are rarely bored.

Nursing has exceptional variety. There is med-surg, OB, peds, critical care. You can work in a hospital, clinic, school, or industry. You can go into home care or private practice. There are opportunities in education, management, and research.

Flexible hours. That's an excellent example of disguising a problem as an opportunity. If you check the fine print, you will find flexible hours means working nights, weekends, holidays, and summer vacations. But flexible hours is a strong selling point, especially for women. Women today are still held accountable for most child care and household tasks. In addition, they are expected to want more than a job, they are expected to pursue a career. The only way women can do that is via flexible hours.

Money! Starting salaries are excellent and in 1995 the average nurse was making over $40,000 a year. Some were making twice that amount.

And it is personally rewarding. Nursing has intangible rewards that cannot be matched in many other occupations. One of the things employees in any field crave most is "meaningful work." Nursing has that in spades, but sometimes we forget. We need to remind ourselves and each other of the good things about nursing.

Some other "convincing" reasons include:

The ever-popular "meet-and-marry-a-doctor."
"Challenging! Nursing pushes me to my limits."
"It's good training for motherhood."
"You don't need a large wardrobe to work."
"It's a good profession to fall back on—sort of like Social Security (and just as solvent?)."

If you are an optimist or an opportunist, you might see this as an excellent time to enter the nursing profession.

"The *future* in nursing looks good!"
"You can only move *up!*"

Those viewing nursing most favorably fall into two categories: unemployed nurses and nurses who hold health care jobs outside of hospitals. Many view nursing as an excellent stepping-stone to more flexible, creative, autonomous jobs inside and outside the health care system.

Lately there is some evidence that nursing may once again be losing its foremost point of appeal—"You can always get a job." If the economic recession/depression of the early 1990s does nothing else, it has managed to ease the nurse shortage. Part-time nurses began asking to work full-time as their husbands' jobs were threatened or lost. Nurses who hadn't darkened the door of a hospital in years suddenly enrolled in refresher courses and signed on to work.

Educators and recruiters may view this turn of events as either a problem or an opportunity, but the pressure is off. As long as the demand for nurses exceeded the supply, the profession was pressured to step up the manufacturing process. The advent of associate degree nursing programs was one result. No matter how many new nurses graduated each year, institutions seemed to gobble them up and cry out for more. In our haste to manufacture the right quantity, some fear we have sacrificed our commitment to quality.

Perhaps in 1999 there will be a great nurse recall. Automobile manufacturers do it all the time. Perhaps nurses, like cars, will run the risk of being labeled "unsafe at any speed." We will have to scrap them or take them back to the factory to be rebuilt.

The idea of making the baccalaureate degree the entry level into professional practice is an idea whose time has come . . . and gone . . . and perhaps come again. During this respite when we are not driven to manufacture vast quantities of nurses, we have the opportunity to reevaluate and, if necessary, revamp nursing education.

Right now, to become a nurse you must successfully survive an educational process lasting anywhere from 2 to 5 years. The fact that it takes some people twice as long as others to become nurses causes conflict inside the profession and confusion outside the profession. Our indecisiveness is embarrassing.

Since we have never delineated exactly what services a nurse will provide, we must guess at what she needs to know to be equal to the task. And the "task" of nursing seems to encompass everything from providing the most elementary physical care to performing the most sophisticated research.

Attempting to define nursing, one man wrote, "Nursing is what nurses do. And nurses *do everything!*" The expectation that a nurse must be a "jack-of-all-trades and master of 'some'" is unrealistic. No wonder nurses are anxious. No wonder we are obsessed with education. How do you educate someone to "do everything"?

Ars longa, vita brevis.

Translation: "The life so short, the craft so long to learn."

Although encouraging a commitment to lifelong learning may be desirable, nurses seem to have an unhealthy compulsion to educate, reeducate, and continually educate. Perhaps our educational goal is so unclear we don't recognize it when we reach it.

Few students are adequately counseled about the strengths and limitations of the various nursing education programs available. Their choice is not determined by past performance, future potential, or long-range career goals. Most often it is determined by whichever program is quickest, cheapest, or closest to home.

For decades problems of educational mobility have plagued nursing. For a while the career-ladder concept seemed promising. That concept is based on the assumption that there is a common information core that can be built on at any future time. Logically, with additional education and experience, an able nurse's aide should be able to move up to the practical nurse level, and a practical nurse should be able to move up to the associate degree level and become a registered nurse.

This ladder works well through the associate degree level. At that point, halfway up the educational ladder, many nurses seem to be stuck. Those wishing to pursue their studies for a bachelor of science in nursing degree are essentially told they have to start at the bottom and make the whole climb again.

One very successful director of nursing (a diploma graduate) shared her difficulties when she tried to pursue a BSN degree. At the state university she was told her previous experience and education were worth a sum total of nine college credits. Angry and frustrated, she turned away from the school of nursing and is now completing her master's in business administration.

When a hospital diploma program and a private college merged to offer both a generic BSN program and an external degree BSN program (one that would be offered off campus at different locations throughout the state), the response was overwhelming. Before the program officially opened, the college had received 14,000 requests for information, and 3500 nurses visited the campus personally.

In spring 1982 I was hired to set up an associate degree nursing program for a small community college in Oregon. While I was busily laying the foundation for the new program, the Oregon State Board of Nursing made a motion to require the baccalaureate degree for entry into professional practice by 1990. That motion caused an uproar.

Overnight two camps formed: those who supported associate degree nursing education and those who supported baccalaureate nursing education. In hopes of minimizing polarization, nurse educators quickly formed a special interest group consisting of the deans and directors of the state's various nursing programs.

Dialogue was spirited. If the ADN backers were guilty of trying to teach their students to *do* everything, then the BSN backers were guilty of trying to teach their students to *be* everything. Supporters of baccalaureate education campaigned for one level of nursing practice—professional. Supporters of associate degree education campaigned for two levels of nursing practice—technical and professional.

In one important area the ADN educators had a distinct advantage. They knew the limits of their graduates. Their scope of practice had already been carefully defined and published. Feeling the role, education, identification, licensure, and employment of the "technical" nurse were well established, they challenged the BSN educators to address the same issues for the "professional" nurse.

During these lively exchanges, the nurse educators discovered that they had more in common than any one of them had dared hope. All recognized this was not a "we-they" problem but an "us" problem. The group set about changing the problem into an opportunity. Resolution was no longer a dream but a goal.

Although early discussions picked at whether registered nurses *should* or *must* have baccalaureate degrees, later discussions focused on the real questions: who, what, when, where, why, how, and how much?

When college presidents, legislators, and others offered their muscle and advice, they were told this was an intraprofessional problem and the nurses would handle it.

The decision to support one or two levels of nursing education may not be as important as the fact that a decision is made and that nurses make it.

It is now 1996. The "deadline" in Oregon came and went 6 years ago just as it has come and gone in so many states for so many years. The American Nurses Association's position on entry was initiated in 1965. Thirty years have passed and only *one* state has managed to make it a reality. In June of 1995, ANA reaffirmed its commitment. Nurses, this may be our last chance to establish a profession. Let's not blow it.

Margaretta Styles* and a covey of her graduate students, writing in *Nursing Outlook,* have this to say:

> Ironically, the U.S., with the most highly developed system of university nursing education, may eventually be left in the wake of a higher universal standard for licensure or registration. Even today, we are one of the few countries that require only two years of nursing education for the coveted RN ("first level") title and license.

And later in the article:

> To be quite blunt . . . Despite all of the protections promised through grandfathering, pathways to educational mobility, and other means, the entry movement tends to be perceived by many to be "demoting" and affecting the lives and livelihoods of hundreds of thousands of RNs who do not possess the education to meet the proposed standard.

Just as parents want the best for their children, you and I should want the best for our offspring: the next generation of nurses. Changing the entry into practice has nothing to do with the past. It has to do with the future.

Most of the nurses reading this book will have felt the anguish and frustration of those "hundreds of thousands of RNs." Most of us began our careers without a baccalaureate education. Many of us painstakingly completed our education. It was brutal. The rest of us are guilt-ridden because we haven't completed our education. All of us are angry.

Do we want the same misery visited on the next generation?

---

*Styles, Margaretta, et al.: "Entry: A new approach," *Nursing Outlook* 39(5):200–203, Sept.-Oct. 1991.

A popular definition of insanity is doing the same things over and over again and expecting different results.

In "a call to action" at the conclusion of the article, Styles, who is proposing that we set up a system for national voluntary certification of professional nurses, writes:

> It sometimes seems that our professional character is a paradoxical mix of high idealism and unchecked egalitarianism. In many ways, this combination serves us well in nursing practice. However, in professional matters it often causes us to pursue the impossible or surrender to paralysis.

This is our profession. It is our right and responsibility to determine how future nurses will be created, licensed, and utilized. If we fail to make these decisions, they will be made for us.

Chapter 4

Procuring and Keeping Nurses

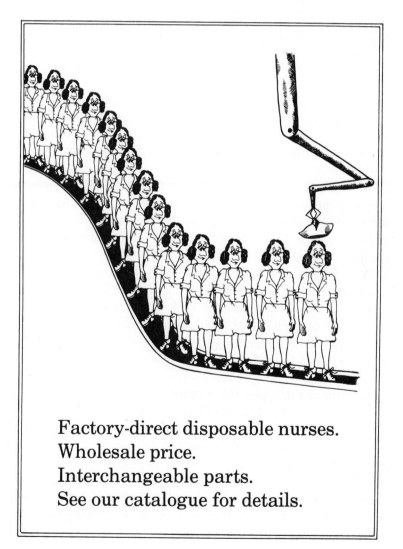

Factory-direct disposable nurses.
Wholesale price.
Interchangeable parts.
See our catalogue for details.

LET'S talk about headhunters. Not the kind you find in the wilds of Borneo but the sophisticated kind. The ones who hunt topnotch professionals and outstanding executives. Corporations pay such headhunters handsome sums because they know the value of having the right person in the right job. They also know the cost of having the wrong person.

Unfortunately, when it comes to filling nursing vacancies, hospitals don't hunt heads, they hunt *herds!* Large, docile herds of nurses who will meander in, graze awhile, and then move on to greener pastures.

When it comes to nurses, hospitals have always been more interested in quantity than quality. That's because they can count better than they can think.

There are several reasons why hospitals don't engage in headhunting. One is that nurses are not thought to need very good heads. They are literally hired hands. In fact, many who employ and manage nurses prefer nurses who are not very "head strong." Another reason is that headhunting looks expensive. Hospitals are penny-wise and pound-foolish institutions. Third, luring an outstanding nurse away from her present employer by offering her more money is too radical an idea. It flies in the face of one of hospitaldom's oldest beliefs: nurses are interchangeable. Besides, if the herd got wind of it, they might stampede.

Traditionally hospitals have been content to make do with whatever nurses they had on hand. If they didn't happen to have enough on hand, they sat back and waited for some to wander in.

Until the new "stock" arrived, the old staff was prodded to work longer and harder: take on double shifts, forego days off, and increase patient loads. Under the strain many loyal, long-term nurse employees resigned.

The herd-management mentality persisted: "Well, that's just the way nurses are. They don't stay in any hospital very long. They are always looking for greener pastures." Even when the nurse shortage became critical, hospitals balked at making their own grasses greener.

The nurse shortage escalated. Soon even hospitals with religious affiliations didn't have a prayer when it came to acquiring the nurses they needed. Nurses were staying away from hospitals in droves. Desperation increased.

Hospitals tried to maintain their high standards for hiring nurses: "If it's walking, breathing, and licensed—hire it!" As the shortage wore on, they began settling for two out of three.

One vacationing nurse happened upon a lovely little community. She was so attracted to the spot that she called the hospital and the two nursing homes located there. All three tried to hire her over the phone, sight unseen!

Another nurse decided to go on a round of interviews just to see what else might be available in her city. During the first few moments of one interview she was asked if she had brought a uniform with her. At another institution she was asked if she could begin work that evening.

Clinging to the belief that it was more important to find new nurses than to hold their own, hospitals poured money into newspaper and journal advertisements. They took out bigger, better, and longer-running classified ads. One hospital laughingly became known as "Our Lady of the Perpetual Want Ad."

But nurses had become more astute at reading those ads. We knew that "competitive salaries" meant they paid the exact same salary as every other institution in the area. We knew "challenging positions" meant twice the work for the same salary. In short, the more elaborate the ad, the lower the salary and the heavier the work load.

Reluctantly hospitals began to relinquish another of their most cherished beliefs: nurses are disposable. Besides attracting new nurses, they realized the necessity of keeping their old ones. Resisting the obvious (raising salaries, increasing fringe benefits, and improving working conditions), they offered minor prizes, gimmicks, and gags: laundry service, free parking, all the coffee you could drink. Eventually those Cracker Jack prizes grew into cash bounties, new cars for night nurses, and trips to Hawaii. (When they were just on the verge of having to offer something substantial, the entire economy of the United States collapsed in the early 1980s and the shortage was solved . . . at least temporarily. By the late 1980s the shortage had resurfaced with a vengeance. Substantive gains were made. In the early 1990s the economy collapsed again. When the shortage rebounds all indications are it will be the most severe nurse shortage ever. Why? Because we are an aging population.)

The recent nurse shortages spawned countless theories, excuses, committees, commissions, and studies. The first major nurse shortage also spawned a new position in many hospitals: nurse recruiter.

A nurse was singled out and given responsibility for solving the shortage at her particular hospital. Often she knew nothing of public relations, advertising, promotion, marketing, or personnel management. She was simply appointed and told to recruit.

At the height of the last nurse shortage, I conducted a little experiment. I called all the hospitals in a large city and asked for their nurse recruiter. Using my sister's name and address, I told them I was moving into their city and wanted to find a job. I asked if there was anything special I should know about their hospital. I also requested any brochures or information they could send to help me learn about their facility.

I had created a thumbnail sketch of my experience, education, and interests so I would be consistent in what I shared with each recruiter. (That's not easy when you're a psych nurse who is trying to pass for a med-surg nurse.)

To my surprise—and relief—not one recruiter asked me any questions about my personal or professional life. There was no attempt to engage me in conversation. They didn't ask me why I was moving to their city, what I had done professionally, how I had been educated, or what my interests were.

Few had any response to my question, "Is there anything special about your hospital? Is there something that sets it apart from the rest?" After some thought they might mention that they were a teaching-research facility or had a burn unit.

The only hospital that had no recruiter connected me immediately with an assistant director of nursing. She had a ready response to the above questions. Yes, they had something that set them apart. They had an all-RN staff and practiced primary care. Their turnover rate was only 5% a year, and they had a waiting list of nurses who wanted to come and work for them.

Isn't it fascinating that her information packet was the first to arrive? The nonrecruiter, who already had nurses waiting, sent me the requested information first class. Within 48 hours her brochures and application forms were in my hand.

Most of the mailings arrived within 7 days. There were a few stragglers, and one dawdling recruiter took 16 days to deliver any information.

The contents of the packets varied widely. Again, to my surprise, not one included a personal note or anything signed by the recruiter. There were no friendly overtures; no helpful hints to aid in my relocation; no maps or information on housing, schools, or neighborhoods. Nothing. Two recruiters, and I use the term loosely, sent application forms but absolutely no information about their hospitals, not even a picture postcard!

At a time when hospitals were reporting nurse turnover rates ranging from 40% to 100%, you can quickly see what an economic advantage the hospital with a 5% rate enjoyed. The cost of replacing nurses is staggering.

The cost of recruiting, orienting, and bringing *one* new nurse up to speed can be staggering. According to an article in *Nursing Economics**, estimates range from $1,280 to $50,000! These estimates include direct and indirect costs: advertising, temporary nurses, overtime, lost revenues, orientation, training, decreased productivity, and termination.

An example used in that article included an average cost per turnover of $12,147. If your institution employs 500 nurses and has a 40% turnover rate, they are replacing 200 nurses a year at an estimated cost of $2,429,400! It really pays to keep turnover rates down.

To gain insight into what attracts and holds nurses, I began using the following exercise:

"Your best friend from nursing school has just moved to your community. Give her three convincing reasons why she should come to work for your hospital (agency, clinic, institution)."

1. _____ moral isnt bad _____
2. _____ Camerade is great - encouraging colleges _____
3. _____ growth is optional and wonderfulof achieved _____

When workshop groups are given this assignment, an alarming number of nurses are absolutely stumped. They have to think long and hard. Many barely manage one flimsy reason such as, "Well, we'd be together" or "We could car pool." Others have a single plea: "We need you desperately!"

Among workshop participants in large metropolitan areas, usually one hospital's employees are more vocal and more positive

---

*Jones, Cheryl Bland: Calculating and updating nursing turnover costs, *Nursing Economics,* 10(1):39–45, 1992.

than others. When a particularly complimentary reason crops up like "Our nursing administration is dynamic and supportive," the audience is quick to ask, *"Where do you work!?"*

Public relations departments and personnel recruiters would find their present employees' responses to this simple exercise very enlightening. Every employee reflects both the image and substance of the institution. Each is either a walking warning or a walking advertisement for the facility.

Here are a few responses from employees who are walking-talking warnings:

> "I cannot think of any reason to work for my hospital. I'm beginning to wonder why I work for them. They offer absolutely nothing in the line of opportunity or real advancement."
>
> "Don't come to work here—very unstable—administration does not back you."
>
> "I work at 'Rufus Memorial.' Don't go there. Go to 'St. Ignats.'"

Here are one nurse's tongue-in-cheek reasons:

1. You can earn a tiny bit more money.
2. We can have a few laughs.
3. The doctors are extremely ignorant.

One nurse wrote *five* reasons:

1. Good pay
2. Good hours
3. Excellent opportunity for advancement
4. Really care about each employee
5. Bonuses paid for good attendance

That sounds great until you read her final note: "These are fictitious. I'm not employed. But if I could find an employer who would offer any of the above, I'd join the work force again!"

Perhaps the saddest comment, by virtue of its frequency, is, "Our hospital is no worse than any other." Think about it. Does your employer strive for excellence or do only the minimum to prevent slipping from a second-rate to a third-rate hospital?

When discussing reasons to work for an employer, the comments that draw the most audience interest are those related to supportive administrators who listen to suggestions and encourage creativity and autonomy.

Here are some of the reasons listed by employees who are happy to recommend their employers to their best friends:

"Supportive nursing administration"
"Good educational opportunities"
"Lots of intelligent, informed people"
"Friendly"
"Fair"
"Compassionate"
"Time-and-a-half on weekends"
"Trend-setter"
"Computerized system"
"No rotating shifts"
"Superb patient care"
"Open to suggestions"
"Convenient location"
"Small-town atmosphere"
"Support for inventive ideas"
"Flexible schedules"
"Excellent salaries"
"Wonderful fringe benefits"
"Opportunities for personal growth"
"Challenging work"
"State-of-the-art equipment"
"Variety of positions"
"Newest and largest"
"Autonomy of practice"
"Job security"
"Encourages creativity"
"Allows ingenious people to produce"
"Great colleagues"
"Best hospital in town!"

Go back through that list and circle those descriptive phrases that apply to your hospital or employer. Jot down any other reasons to work for your employer here:

_____

_____

_____

If your list is a little thin, it's not unusual.

When it came to courting and keeping nurses, hospitals were notoriously cheap. Some even begrudged "spending" a thank-you on their nurses. Their no-deposit-no-return management style eventually proved their undoing. They refused to invest an extra nickel in their nurses, and their nurses stopped returning.

Turnover rates went from inconvenient to intolerable because turning over was the only way nurses could better their position. As long as a nurse stayed loyal to her employer, she was likely to be stuck on the wrong shift, on the wrong unit, and at a salary often lower than that of a newly hired nurse.

Lo and behold, nurses were not immune to overwork and impervious to insults and abuse. Loyal nurses began to demand loyalty from their employers. Nickels spent on recruitment had to be matched by nickels spent on retention efforts.

Hospitals began investing nickels in nurses. They spent one nickel on salaries, another on fringe benefits. They hired nurse recruiters and financed toll-free phone numbers, open houses, convention booths, fancy advertisements, and press parties.

They spent a few nickels on other inventive incentives to attract and hold their nurses, including such things as free prescription drugs, free tax service, free coffee, cafeteria discounts, garden patches, memberships in recreation facilities at reduced prices, social events, jogging tracks, on-site child care, awards for good attendance, monetary bonuses for unused sick leave, and short-term cash advances on future earnings.

Seattle's Virginia Mason Hospital sponsors a Nurse Recognition Day. Peers vote for outstanding nurses. Winners are not only honored at a party, they are given a day off with pay.

This hospital also had difficulty keeping experienced critical care nurses on nights. Most nurses work their way off nights, leaving that undesirable shift to inexperienced nurses. However, night nurses have little backup or support. Growing concerns about patient safety sparked a creative scheduling plan.

Critical-care night nurses could work 7 on and 7 off. Their 7 on consisted of 4 nights on, 1 off, 2 nights on. The next 7 they were off. They could ski midweek, take a minivacation, work on their thesis, or volunteer time with church or community organizations without worrying about their schedule.

In addition, if the nurse was willing to work 1 or 2 nights on her week off, the hospital paid her *double* her hourly rate. It is no more expensive than hiring an agency nurse, and the hospital got a high-quality, experienced nurse. No more pigs in a poke. I had never seen such happy night nurses. They were handsomely rewarded financially and they felt like they had 26 weeks of vacation a year. Instead of trying to work their way off nights, CCRNs were trying to work their way onto nights!

Some of the best incentives to stay with an employer don't cost a cent. Courtesy and compliments are free. They are also highly contagious. Introduce them in your hospital, and they will spread like wildfire.

A nurse manager in Illinois told me one of her goals was to compliment at least 12 people a day. To keep track, she put 12 pennies in her left pocket. Every time she gave a compliment, she transferred a penny to her right pocket. When all of the pennies were in her right pocket, she knew she had met her goal.

The best-selling *One Minute Manager* suggested catching people doing things right. One midwestern hospital operationalized that idea by placing "praise boxes" throughout the facility. Next to the brightly colored boxes were "praise coupons," which had lines for the date, the name of the person you saw going a bit above and beyond the call of duty, a brief description of what they were doing, and a place for your signature.

At the end of the month, the coupons would be gathered. A copy was put in the person's file while he or she received the original. An employee of the month was selected. That person got to have any parking space she wanted for the next 30 days and a dinner served to her and a companion by the department head of her choice. The "waiter" would drape a towel over the arm and solicitously bow and scrape.

After 12 months they selected an employee of the year. There was a luncheon, a plaque, and a check for $100.

Initially the boxes were rarely used. In fact, you might have been selected employee of the month because you were the only one who got a coupon! But management never let on. They made a big production out of the monthly event. After 4 or 5 months, the praise boxes began to fill up. Housekeepers were praising doctors, doctors were praising nurses, nurses were praising dietitians, and dietitians were praising housekeepers. The entire atmosphere of the organization changed. After 3 years the "Praise Program" was still extremely popular.

At first a staff developer at a California hospital strongly resisted the suggestion that nurses nominate a "Doctor of the Year" as part of the annual Nurses' Week celebration. She thought Nurses' Week should only honor nurses. Her staff nurses, however, outvoted her.

Today she is delighted they did. The Doctor of the Year Award has empowered nurses and greatly improved doctor-nurse relationships. The essays written to nominate the doctors are published by the in-house newsletter.

Each year the number of nominees, the mystery, and the excitement have grown. Dozens of doctors now attend the Nurses' Week banquet to see who the winner will be. The chosen doctor then shares the stage with the Nurse of the Year.

Too often compliments, like eulogies, are saved for the dearly departed. Until a nurse retires or resigns, no one bothers to tell her how much she is appreciated. Many insist if they had known how much they would be missed, they might not have quit.

When nurses are asked to share the latest compliment they received in the workplace, the lack of examples is disheartening. When asked to share the latest compliment they *gave* in the workplace, the silence is eloquent.

There are some notable exceptions, like the nurse who found an envelope taped to her locker. In it was a letter from the director of nurses letting her know how much her efforts were appreciated. It contained specific examples of how she had helped patients, families, and colleagues and expressed the hope that she would remain on staff for a long time to come. It brought tears to her eyes. (Note: a copy of that letter was placed in the nurse's permanent file.)

The director's action so impressed me that I telephoned her the following day. I thought she should know the impact her action had on that workshop group. She was delighted to get positive feedback. Her letter-writing campaign was a new venture inspired by her motto: "Happy nurses mean happy patients."

Each unit within the hospital also has responsibility for recruitment and retention. One especially hectic medical-surgical unit kept demanding more nurses. The recruiter tried to service them but every nurse she sent was chewed up and spit out in rapid order. Each lasted only a few months. During exit interviews they told painful tales of being harrassed and, worse yet, ignored. Most not only left the unit, they left the hospital.

When the recruiter talked with the veteran nurses on the unit, they insisted they had no time to babysit the newcomers. It was a sink-or-swim operation. The recruiter should stop sending them inexperienced losers.

The recruiter agreed to stop. In fact, she told them she would not send them *any* new nurses until they developed a detailed plan to help newcomers adjust to the unit.

Faced with that ultimatum, the med-surg nurses put their heads together. They identified the best nurses to function as mentors and preceptors. The new nurse would work in tandem with an experienced nurse—one known for patience, knowledge, and understanding. They hosted a "welcome" party for the newcomer. They developed a handout describing the unit and providing a thumbnail sketch of every nurse currently employed there, including the nurse's particular area of expertise and home phone numbers. The new nurse was encouraged to call if she had questions. At 1 month, the head nurse took the newcomer out for a celebration luncheon, at 6 months the staff shared an anniversary cake, and at 1 year they presented the "survivor" with a special you-are-one-of-us pin.

Today that unit's turnover rate is almost nil. It has become a model for other units in the hospital that are having difficulty recruiting and retaining good nurses.

The same strategies can be applied to temporary help. Most nurses hate to float. An assistant head nurse on a large surgical unit described the problem this way:

> Float nurses coming to our unit were resentful. They refused to take an assignment unless they were coassigned with a unit nurse. The unit nurses then resented the floats because of the dual assignment, the extra responsibility, and the attitude of the float. They claimed the extra "help" was actually a hindrance.
>
> At a staff conference we came up with the following solution. We decided the float nurse was a guest on our unit and would be treated as such. The unit nurse would buddy with the float. They would work together as a team to accomplish the shared patient care. The choice of break and lunch time would be given to the float nurse as our guest. The coassigned unit nurse would accompany her.

Float nurses could request to be coassigned with a specific unit nurse. Most importantly, a "thank-you" note was sent to the float nurse by her unit nurse. The notes were designed by the unit secretary and copied as needed.

Attitudes changed on both sides. The float and unit nurses got to know each other better. Unit nurses felt special when requested by the float nurse. The float nurse enjoyed the experience and the thank-you notes. Tension went down. Morale went up.

Happy nurses do mean happy patients. What are you doing to keep the nurses on your unit happy?

Penny-pinching institutions should be reminded that the least expensive and most effective recruiting is done by satisfied employees. Happy employees enthusiastically recommend their employer to friends and neighbors, colleagues and classmates. Other successful "recruiters" are satisfied patients, board members, and auxiliary volunteers who sing praises to the professionals they meet.

The most expensive and least effective way to recruit is through classified advertisements, whether they are placed in newspapers, professional journals, or trade magazines. Even using commercial headhunting agencies is more productive and less expensive.

Of course, some ads are more imaginative and more effective than others. Denver General Hospital reduced their RN vacancies from 50 to 6 with a campaign built around the theme "put yourself on the edge of excellence." Instead of the hit-and-miss recruitment programs many hospitals conduct, Denver General analyzed its product, defined target consumers, appraised their competition, and hit the bull's eye.

Ads aimed at herds rarely produce the desired results. Any recruiter worth her salt knows ad campaigns must be directed toward specific targets. A worthy recruiter also knows the best targets.

Nursing students about to enter the labor market for the first time are ready recruits. They should be vigorously courted and eased into their first professional assignment gently. If your facility develops a reputation as a good place to launch a career, you can have the cream of the crop from any nursing school.

If you abuse new graduates, giving them too much too soon,

you will develop a reputation as a bad place to launch a career. The cream of the crop will go elsewhere. You'll get the leftovers.

Other prime targets are people who call or write the hospital for information. They should be given first-class attention. What about nurses who walk in unannounced? Roll out the red carpet! They have made the first move, the next move is yours. First impressions can entice the potential staff member to take a closer look or send them running toward the nearest exit.

The phrase "exit interview" always struck me as a bit silly. In my mind it ranks right up there with "wrongful death," which implies there is a "rightful death."

Since I always thought exit interviews were futile, you can imagine my surprise when a hospital in New Orleans told me they not only did exit interviews but gave the departing nurse a gift certificate. Crazy? Yes, crazy like a fox.

A nurse may leave your organization for any number of personal or professional reasons. By giving the gift certificate, the hospital was saying, "Look, we know the grass is always greener on the other side of the fence. And we wish you all the best. However, if things don't work out quite as you'd hoped or planned, we would love to welcome you back. There will always be a light on in the window here at Our Lord Have Mercy for you."

Flipping through the pages of an in-flight magazine, I saw an article titled "Two-Timers." It wasn't the juicy article I thought it would be. It was about recruitment. The theme of the article was that the best place to find new employees was among your former employees. It pays to keep in touch and track them down. It pays to part friends.

When the nurse shortage abates, do hospitals disband their recruitment and retention efforts? The smart ones don't. They continue their efforts because they know that their survival is linked both to the quantity and quality of nurses they hire.

Hospitals no longer have a blank check to cover their expenses and ensure their future. Cost containment is imperative. Institutions that are not fiscally fit will die. As has already been discussed, the cost of replacing nurses is prohibitive. Dollars invested in successful retention programs will pay for themselves a hundredfold.

Just as hospitals cannot afford to replace nurses, they cannot afford to hire the wrong nurses. Herds of nurses just passing through (floats, rentals, and novices) can spell financial disaster. Today, more than ever, things have to be done right the first time. With the advent of DRGs, a high-quality staff will pay for itself. A low-quality staff will put the hospital out of business.

As hospitals scramble for survival, the demand for herds will be down and heads up!

Diagnoses Related Groups cost containment

Chapter 5

Prolonging Professional Life

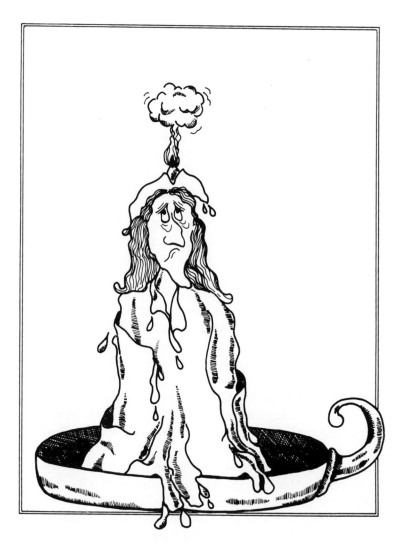

FOR years Sally had worked at a large state institution. The staffing was poor, the equipment archaic, the leadership lethargic, and the patients chronic.

For several months she had been feeling increasingly irritable and fatigued. Her optimism had been slowly replaced by a nagging pessimism. She had begun to question the institution's priorities, psychiatry's usefulness, the patients' progress, nursing's future, and her own competence.

Only two things kept her on the job: a fading sense of duty and overwhelming inertia. When she tried to discuss her feelings with colleagues, they were either too busy or too frustrated themselves to listen.

A classic case of burnout, wouldn't you say? You and I both know all the signs and symptoms. Burnout is easy to spot—in other people.

Unfortunately, the onset is so insidious and gradual, the person with the "disease" is often the last to know. That's why it is so important to have good friends, colleagues, and supervisors who can sense trouble and send help before burnout extinguishes your career.

In Sally's case burnout was cured in a dramatic and highly unorthodox way. Near midnight, after a particularly trying shift, she left the hospital alone. Walking through the parking lot, she was jumped by a mugger.

She beat the bejeebers out of him!

She kicked, clawed, punched, and generally walloped him. All the time she was shrieking at the top of her lungs. When help came running, they had to pull *her* off him.

Later she compared the mugger's attack to shock therapy. It jolted her out of apathy and into action. In those few moments, all her pent-up anger and frustration were released.

Suddenly energized, she began to evaluate her professional future. She realized she wasn't doing anyone a favor by staying in her present position.

Three weeks later she took a new job in a community mental health center. Her energy, optimism, and creativity returned. Once again she began enjoying work instead of enduring it.

"Enduring" work is one warning signal of impending burnout. Other signs and symptoms might include:

Irritability	No sense of purpose	Smoking more
Impatience	Bitching	Drinking more
Fatigue	Boredom	Eating more
Exhaustion	Malaise	Feeling guilty
Depression	Whining	Dreading work
Cynicism	Weeping	Apathy
Pessimism	Poor concentration	Loneliness
Loss of idealism	Indecisiveness	Uncooperativeness
Carelessness	Feeling helpless	Paralyzed creativity
Playing hooky	Feeling powerless	Denial
Being tardy	Callousness	Rationalization
Aches and pains		Insomnia

Usually, before you burn out, you have to burn up. Anger, frustration, and righteous indignation are not uncommon predecessors. Your professional survival depends on what you do with that anger. Anger is energy. Channeled properly, changes can be made and burnout averted.

If you absorb the anger instead of harnessing it, the result is depression. There is no energy in depression. There is only resignation: "What's the use? Who cares? I give up."

Who are the people most susceptible to burnout? The best and the brightest. Hardworking idealists. Perfectionists.

Which jobs lend themselves most to burnout? Jobs in which constant high performance is required. Jobs in which expectations are unclear or unrealistic. Jobs in which workers have little control over what they do or how they do it. Demanding, stressful, people-related jobs. Jobs that couple overwhelming responsibility with powerlessness. Jobs that offer little financial reward, recognition, or appreciation.

Nursing fits the description. Nurses are prime candidates for burnout.

Although information about burnout is important, knowledge alone will not prevent it any more than knowledge will prevent disease. Knowledge is a tool. Unless you pick up the tool and use it to change your professional lifestyle, it is worthless.

If you want to save your professional life, here are a half-dozen suggestions:

Learn to Pace Yourself

Many burnout victims approach their career as though it were a hundred-yard dash instead of a multi-mile marathon. Quickly caught up in the frenzy around them, they dash from crisis to crisis.

Perhaps they really believe that by working harder and longer, they can get everyone well. Then, and only then, will they sit down and take a break.

Professionals like that never get a break. They just get broken.

Take Care of Yourself

If you don't take care of yourself, no one else will. Eat right. Get enough rest. Exercise regularly. Be kind to yourself.

Fence off a few minutes each day just to reflect and dream in solitude. Forget the boss, patients, spouse, children, in-laws. Take time to renew yourself physically, mentally, emotionally, and spiritually. Private time is not a luxury. It's a necessity.

Take care of yourself or you won't be around to take care of others.

I heard of a nurse who was doing her master's thesis on what she was calling "the nurse's retention syndrome." This was the voluntary suppression of the urge to void for between 8 to 12 hours a day. She figured every nurse had a bladder the size of a basketball because nurses do such important work, they can't take time for lunch, or for a break, or even for a quick trip to the bathroom!

We are so busy caring for others, we often neglect our own health. We preach good health to patients but we don't practice it ourselves.

The staff developer in a Georgia hospital wanted to encourage wellness. She devised a simple walking program that she called "Fun Fit." She marked off 1-mile and 2-mile paths outside on hospital grounds. For days when the weather was gruesome, she plotted 1-mile and 2-mile courses right inside the hospital.

She sent around a sign-up sheet expecting about 40 nurses to register. Well, almost 400 nurses registered! The fitness program became a third of her job description. Before long the walking program expanded to include swimming, golf, tennis, jazzercise, etc. The next thing she knew nurses were teaming up for friendly competition. For example, nurses working with diabetic patients all wore matching T-shirts that said "Sugar Bears." Soon people were coming from other departments asking if they could join the program. The administrator wanted in on the fun. He helped with awards and prizes. The fitness craze swept through the entire institution.

Learn to Leave Work Behind

Don't let work preempt your personal life. Socialize. Protect your family time.

Be aware of how work can contaminate your personal life. Alice is a good example of this problem. She had worked almost 3 years in neonatal intensive care. Originally she and her husband, Steve, had planned to save for a house and then have children. They both loved children.

Financially secure and house in hand, Steve was surprised when Alice suddenly refused to have children. Actually, it wasn't a sudden decision at all. It wasn't even a conscious decision. The daily dose of pain, death, and disability of her tiny patients and their distraught parents had subtly taken its toll. Alice was no longer anxious to have children. She was terrified.

The marriage nearly collapsed before Alice got the help she needed. Fortunately, the hospital had an excellent psychiatrist available to the staff and an active peer-counseling program. A change of assignment and some intense, individual therapy helped Alice regain a healthy perspective.

Today, with two thriving children of her own, Alice is thinking of returning to neonatal ICU. She feels her maturity and positive personal experiences have made her strong enough to again tackle that difficult assignment.

Some experts think non–work-related activities are the key to preventing burnout. That poses a special problem for women whose professional duties are often an extension and refinement of what they do at home: cook, clean, comfort, etc.

To effectively separate your personal and professional life, you may need some decompression time between work and home. Jog, dance, garden, swim, or sauna. Participate in activities that clear your mind and refresh your spirit. Don't be surprised if you have to *work* at relaxation.

Activate Assertiveness Skills

Take the initiative. Make choices not excuses. Ask for what you need. Ask for what you want.

Say no to double shifts, 7-day stretches, and duties sloughed by impertinent physicians and uncooperative colleagues.

Say yes to the nursing activities you thoroughly enjoy. Make good use of the 80/20 principle by remembering that 80 percent of the pleasure you derive from nursing will come from completing 20 percent of your duties.

Identify the duties that give you the most satisfaction. One way to do this is to complete the following sentence in as many ways as possible:

"I feel very satisfied when I leave work knowing _____

_____

_____."

Here are some examples from other nurses:

"I feel very satisfied when I leave work knowing . . .
I handled interpersonal problems tactfully."
the families' needs have been met."
the charts are complete."
the utility rooms are clean."
the medications were given on time."
I listened carefully."
the patients are better informed."
I learned something new."
I used my knowledge and skill to the best of my ability."
I was super efficient."
the next shift has the information and supplies needed."
I have made *one* patient more comfortable."

You will never *find* time to do the things you enjoy most in nursing. You have to *make* time for them. Maximize your professional satisfaction by indulging in your favorite nursing activities daily. Satisfied nurses don't burn out.

⚕

Optimize Time Management

Simplify. Set priorities. Delegate.

Clarify your values. Set goals and direct your activities toward their achievement.

Spend time wisely. Invest it. Don't squander it on people or activities unless they are really important to you.

Everyone wants more time. Unfortunately, you already have all the time there is—168 hours a week. No more and no less. We are all exactly equal in this one regard.

The reason some people are able to accomplish so much more than others is that they have learned to delegate. Here are some tips for effective delegation:

1. Focus on *RESULTS*. Too often we focus on efforts. Who will put in the blood, sweat, and tears? When the desired outcome is clearly and realistically defined, it becomes easier to delegate.
2. Share complete information. Give the person what he or she needs to know to be successful.
3. Be willing to give real authority and decision-making power. This may be why nurses have so much trouble delegating. We perceive ourselves as having so little real authority and decision-making power, we are afraid that if we delegate we will lose what little we have. The opposite is true. The more you learn to delegate, the broader your authority and power base.
4. Don't procrastinate. Delegate now! How many times have you thought that it was just easier or faster to do things yourself? It still means *YOU* have to do it. Your time is taken doing things your spouse, your children, your co-workers, your patients could have done for themselves. How will they ever learn if you don't allow them to try? Pick one chore and delegate it today. Don't put it off. Practice delegation until you get good at it.
5. Choose your delegate. Consciously assess that person's skill, experience, and attitude. Talk with her or him about the project. Discuss goals, priorities, deadlines, suggestions. You may need to adjust the current workload so your delegate has time

to do a good job. Give action tips to help promote success.

6. Follow up. There should be some controls and checkpoints, but I don't mean you should spy on or hover over the person. Once you delegate, it is no longer any of your business how the job gets done.

7. Back the delegate to the hilt. Occasionally there is a tattletale or troublemaker in the group. If gossip or complaints come your way, tell the weasels that if they have a problem they should talk candidly with the delegate. After all, the delegate has full authority and decision-making power.

8. GIVE CREDIT. TAKE BLAME! This is a most important step. Sometimes I can almost see a nurse thinking, "Hey, this delegation stuff might not be so bad. If I delegate and the person does a good job, I can take the credit. If she screws up, she gets the blame."

No, the opposite is true. If I delegate and the person does a good job, she gets all the credit. If she screws up, I take the heat because I'm the one who chose her.

If you follow this advice, the next time you have something to delegate, you will have lots of volunteers. If you don't, the next time your volunteers will all disappear.

Respect Your Humanness

You're only human. That's your greatest strength and your greatest weakness.

Resist unrealistic demands from within or without. Don't succumb! Don't be a dodo (Dead On Duty Overdose).

Scheduling practices that changed brand new doctors "from paragons of bright-eyed, enthusiastic energy into a state of exhausted, head-nodding stupor" alarmed Dr. Martin Moore-Ede. He has spent most of his professional life at Harvard Medical School and its spinoff, The Institute for Circadian Physiology, studying the "human clock" and all the ramifications of fatigue.

He finds it especially ironic that "the medical profession—the profession that ought to be most knowledgeable about human physiology and its limitations—adopted work practices that lead to breakdown of the human machine."

Do yourself a favor. Get your hands on a copy of his book, *The Twenty-Four Hour Society* (Addison-Wesley Publishing Co., 1993).

He's an excellent writer who will hold you spellbound as he examines the cost of human breakdown from the Exxon Valdez to Chernobyl to airplane disasters and traffic fatalities.

The next time you see a headline about medical malpractice you'll remember him saying, "fatigue and incompetence dance hand in hand."

Dr. Moore-Ede says we treat machines better than the people who operate them.

> People don't release smoke, grind gears, or have pieces fall off; but their equivalents—fatigue, error, injury, and ill health—do result in failure and breakdown.

We expect humans to be totally flexible and completely adaptable. That belief is erroneous, dangerous, and expensive.

Our nonstop world "forces us to operate the human body outside specs crafted by prehistoric experience." The result? Chronic fatigue, sleep deprivation, malaise, mood disorders, indigestion, cardiovascular malfunctions, suicide, chemical dependency, errors, accidents, and death. The cost? Billions of dollars!

Every nurse who's ever done nights or rotated shifts will find the section on "shift maladaptation syndrome" fascinating. It scientifically confirms what your gut told you long ago. Both can be hazardous to your health.

In December 1995 Harvard University researchers reported that women who work rotating shifts for 6 years or more face a 50% higher risk of developing heart disease than those who work regular shifts. The findings are based on questionnaires from nearly 122,000 *female registered nurses* who have been participants in the ongoing Nurse's Health Study that began in 1976. According to the lead author of the study, Ichiro Kawachi, those at risk should limit the number of years they do shift work. They should eat a low-fat diet, get their blood pressure checked regularly, and not smoke.

While we can't measure fatigue, we can measure alertness by brain waves and eye movements. Perhaps one day when you show up for work, they'll slap a helmet on you, measure your alertness, and determine whether you're fit for duty. Or they may prescribe "prophylactic napping." Evidently taking a 20-minute nap every 4 hours would help us all run longer and stronger.

Because you're human you will have good days and bad days. You'll have days when you're the most gifted nurse on the planet and other days when you're a total klutz. You'll have days when you are oozing the milk of human kindness and other days when you want to tell a whining patient, "If it's such an emergency, dial 911!"

Burnout is contagious. Look closely at your professional companions. When you leave their company, do you feel refreshed and energized or drained and disillusioned?

Andrea, a struggling student nurse, seemed slated for failure. Suddenly she showed great improvement in her academic work. Her clinical performance also improved dramatically.

When her instructor complimented her and asked what had made such a difference, Andrea replied, "Oh, I just switched tables."

Week after week she had sat at the same table in the cafeteria surrounded by students who were also floundering academically and clinically. They spent the lunch hour moaning and complaining.

One noon, during a lengthy tirade by a disgruntled companion, Andrea's attention wandered. She noticed another table where the students were smiling, laughing, and talking excitedly about their experiences. The next day Andrea switched tables.

By the end of the week she began to feel more confident and capable. Soon she no longer questioned her ability to make it in nursing. She was sure she could!

Sometimes you have to fight to save your professional life. Sometimes you have to switch. You may need to switch tables, shifts, units, assignments, hospitals, or jobs. Ideally you won't have to switch careers.

When colleagues begin to flicker and dim, what can you do to help? Encourage them to take a break, minivacation, or mental health day. Listen without being judgmental. Help them identify choices, options, and alternatives. Support their decisions.

Be empathetic. Smile. Say "please" and "thank you." Talk to them. Encourage *esprit de corps*. Invite them to join you at a stress-reduction workshop.

Help them increase their skills in problem solving, time management, and assertiveness. Give positive feedback. Encourage a change in assignments, responsibilities, shifts, or units. Stand up for them. Be there.

Preventive maintenance is as important for people as it is for machinery. Both can burn out if used excessively or improperly.

If you are a manager, whether first-time team leader or well-worn director of nursing, you can help save the professional lives of the people who work for you. Here are some tips:

♦ Assign where they can shine . . . where they can succeed.
♦ Make policies and procedures clear.

- ◆ Clarify role expectations.
- ◆ Define realistic goals for work output.
- ◆ Strengthen problem-solving and time-management skills.
- ◆ Provide an atmosphere of sharing and cohesiveness.
- ◆ Be flexible.
- ◆ Listen.
- ◆ Encourage.
- ◆ Praise.
- ◆ Provide individual counseling or a support group.
- ◆ Encourage growth and development.
- ◆ Individualize orientation.
- ◆ Don't expect perfection.
- ◆ Allow the individual as much control over her own work as possible.
- ◆ Encourage wellness activities.
- ◆ Maintain consistency.
- ◆ Allow direct, honest communication—without reprisals.
- ◆ Infuse with energy and enthusiasm.

If you want to know how to keep your nurse-employees on the job, don't ask the experts, ask your nurses themselves. When I suggest this to managers, they panic. They are sure nurses will immediately ask for more money.

Lack of communication between employers and employees often leads to misinformation and mismanagement. In one study the top six working conditions employees said they wanted were:

1. Interesting work
2. Full appreciation of work done
3. Feeling of being in on things
4. Job security
5. Good pay
6. Promotion and growth

At the same time the top six working conditions their employers *thought* the employees wanted were:

1. Good pay
2. Job security
3. Promotion and growth
4. Good working conditions
5. Interesting work
6. Tactful discipline

If you're still afraid the people who work for you are totally mercenary, try asking them what they want other than higher salaries. I have been asking nurses this question:

> What could your employer do for you, other than offering you more money, to increase your loyalty to the institution and ensure your continued employment?

Although there is some overlapping, most responses fall into six categories: (1) respect, (2) autonomy and opportunity, (3) communication, (4) management style and decision making, (5) education, and (6) financial considerations (suggestions that would cost money). Let me share some quotes with you:

Respect
"Be loyal to me."
"Support me with administration, physicians, and staff."
"Give us the same respect and consideration given doctors."
"Care about my feelings and ideas."
"Treat me fairly."
"Recognize my skills."
"Respect my education and experience."
"Treat me like a professional."
"Let me interview employees for my unit *before* their hiring."
"Provide reserved parking space."
"Stand behind me."
"Trust me."
"Give the nursing staff more say."
"Give praise for a job well done."

Autonomy and opportunity
"Allow me to work freely with ideas."
"Let me follow through on projects I start."
"When you give me a job, let *me* find the best way to do it."
"Make me feel I'm trusted. Don't stand over me all the time."
"Unless I've shown that I'm incompetent, decrease *control* over my activities."
"Give me authority over my own work."
"Provide more support for individual advancement."
"Help me grow in managerial skills."
"Let me know I can advance."

"Allow me freedom to make changes."
"Provide room for intellectual and emotional growth."
"Let me be free to create."
"Promote me!!!"

Communication

"Face-to-face, one-on-one meetings with my supervisor each
    week."
"Listen to my suggestions."
"Keep me informed *before* something changes."
"Encourage us—cheer us on!"
"Give positive feedback . . . occasionally . . . please?"
"Say 'thanks.'"
"Listen. Act when necessary."
"Increase direct, honest communication."
"Talk to *me!*"
"Be truthful."
"Consult us 'little guys' before changing policies."
"Provide more contact with other shifts."

Management style and decision making

"Be fair."
"Lead and guide instead of push."
"Give me bite-sized pieces to work on."
"Be receptive and friendly."
"Support my interests and projects."
"Involve us in management."
"Support my decisions."
"Help problem solve."
"Follow through!"
"Give fair, productive evaluations."
"Less confusion and more organization so I know what my
    job is."
"Be open to suggestions."
"Consistent personnel policies."
"Not on call 24 hours a day, 7 days a week."
"Provide adequate staffing. Not just in numbers but in quality
    as well."
"When it comes to the department I run, let me be the real
    decision maker."

"Have the people who work directly in patient care involved in
   decisions."
"Let us choose the supplies and equipment that we use daily."
"Give me freedom to make decisions appropriate for my position."

Education

"Grant time off for continuing education."
"Provide BSN and MSN classes in hospital."
"Increase educational opportunities."
"Reward academic achievement."
"Allow a schedule flexible enough so I can pursue a degree."
"Unless the hospital is willing to put up the money and free up
   my time, they should get off my back about getting a degree."

Financial considerations

"Raise my salary."
"Increase benefits."
"Fully paid health, dental, and life insurance."
"In-house child care."
"Make three 12-hour shifts full-time."
"No layoffs."
"More overtime."
"Better retirement."
"$100 deductible rather than $300."
"Free tuition."
"Enough equipment to do the job."
"Give us a lounge and cafeteria equal to the one provided for
   doctors."

There were also numerous requests for better hours, more
weekends and holidays off, and flexible schedules. As one nurse put
it, "I'd give anything to get a schedule more congruent with my life."

In conclusion, pause and take a good look at yourself. Professionally speaking, are you alive or just lingering? Are the people
who work with you or for you thriving or barely surviving?

If the quality of your professional life is questionable, prolonging
it may be a grave disservice. There are worse things than death for a
person or a professional. If you have to make a choice, go for quality.

Chapter 6

Profit and Loss

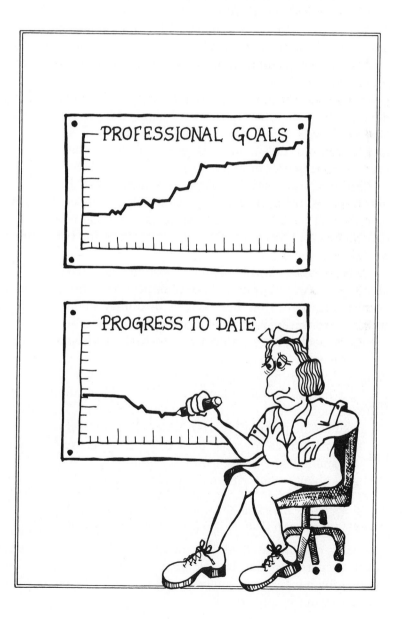

Browsing through a souvenir shop, I spotted a large button that read, *"I'm depressed—no one is after my job."* At the time it was painfully accurate. The nurse shortage was making headlines. While over 100,000 jobs were waiting for nurses to fill them, over 300,000 actively licensed registered nurses were choosing not to work in the health care system.

For a myriad of personal and professional reasons, those nurses had decided they would lose more than they would gain by working. Their *profits* could not adequately compensate them for their *losses*.

For some mysterious reason the laws of supply and demand haven't always applied to nurses. I think the mysterious reason is *Rubber Nurse*. That's the nurse employers can stretch to cover more than one unit or more than one shift. Rubber Nurses (RNs) take on extra patients, extra duties, and extra days.

Believing the nurse shortage is real and not just a figment of low salaries or poor working conditions, Rubber Nurses work longer and harder. Pliable enough to handle everything from orthopedics to obstetrics, RNs can even pass for ICU nurses in a pinch.

When Rubber Nurse begins to lose her elasticity, she is chided about her lack of professional commitment. She is blackmailed with suggestions that her lack of flexibility endangers patients' welfare. Ironically it is her fatigue and her acceptance of assignments exceeding her competence that really endanger patients.

Eventually the paycheck, the pat on the back, the impassioned calls to duty are no longer enough to keep Rubber Nurse bouncing back for more. Stretched beyond her limits, she finally snaps. She bounces right out of her job and/or her profession. The cost of staying has become prohibitive. Her losses exceed her profits.

You and I have invested heavily in nursing. We have put a lot of time, money, and energy into our profession. Many of us never thought about what financial return there would be on such investments.

A 30-year veteran of the nursing profession vividly recalls receiving her first paycheck. When she opened her envelope, she was very disappointed at the amount enclosed. As a student, it never occurred to her to ask about potential salary. When she applied for her first job, she was so excited about being hired, she had not even thought to ask.

Today's women are not that naive. They often consider issues like salary and job security *before* they begin preparing for a particular career. While nursing has its problems, it offers a history of unparalleled job security. And security is what many women value most.

Today's nursing students are *older* and wiser. That 30-year veteran probably began her career at age 21. In 1992 the average age of a newly licensed RN was *33.7* years.

As for money, even the most charitable societies and institutions have begun to admit their survival depends on their ability to turn a profit. They realize profits must not only cover today's expenses but tomorrow's as well. For without sufficient profits there will be no tomorrow.

Profit is not a necessary evil. Profit is simply necessary. When a service or product ceases to be profitable, it ceases to exist.

To survive, any business must be able to cover costs. To *thrive,* a business must do much more. Thriving means having funds for expansion; for education, research, and development; for repairing, replacing, and upgrading equipment; and for meeting rising costs of personnel, goods, and services.

It is almost sacrilegious to link profit and nursing. The thought that we "profit" from others' illnesses and misfortunes seems almost obscene. Yet that is exactly what we do. We fill a vital need, and in return we are paid for our services. *Caring* is our business.

Can nursing accept its need to be profitable? Can you?

Nurses have always been a bit like dethroned royalty—poor but proud. We preferred to focus on tradition, service, sacrifice, duty, and honor. Those were noble words. However, we began to realize that if nursing was to survive and thrive, we would also have to focus on words like "recognition," "respect," "success," and "solvency."

Years ago one nurse put it, "Nursing is a great life but a crummy living." Today, nursing is also a great living.

The average nurse, working full time in acute care, is paid $40,900 a year, according to the 1995 Earnings Survey conducted by *RN* (October, 1995, Vol. 58, Number 10, pp. 48–56). The mean hourly wage was $18.40. In the last 2 years, salaries have risen slowly (about 2%/year), "but still, income is at an all-time high." OR nurses ($19.30) edged out emergency and critical care nursing for the top money slot. Med/surg nurses were the lowest in acute care at $17.70.

A surprising finding was home health nurses' annual income

has almost caught up with acute care nurses. They came in at $40,160, nearly $4400 more than they earned 2 years ago. Nurses in extended care and psychiatric facilities average $36,100. Even with an 8% raise, office nurses make about $4.00 an hour less than hospital nurses. They average $31,120 per year.

There are still nurses who whine about their salaries, thinking they are not making much better than minimum wage. That's so silly. A minimum-wage worker takes home about $10,000. Actually, the *individual* nurse's salary is higher than the average *household* income, even factoring in geographic differences.

While compressed salary scales continue to be a problem, there is lots of evidence that the compression is lifting, shifting, stretching out. We are getting smarter. We realize that if we do not reward our best and our brightest—nurses who invest in higher education, who take on more and more responsibility, and who stay loyal to our institutions—we will lose these people. And there may be no one to replace them.

In the past, loyalty to a health care institution was rarely rewarded and often penalized. Taught that discussing salaries was "unprofessional," many experienced nurses were slow to discover their salaries were actually less than those of newly employed, inexperienced nurses.

At the height of the last nurse shortage in the 1980s, the Colorado legislature agreed to raise entry-level salaries to attract much-needed new nurses. Novices were soon being hired at salaries exceeding those of loyal, long-term nurse employees, not to mention those of their head nurses. The legislators seemed genuinely surprised by the uproar that followed.

Ten or twelve years ago it was not uncommon for an experienced nurse to make only 5% more than a totally inexperienced nurse. One new graduate went to work in the same hospital where her mother had been a nurse for 15 years. They were shocked to discover her starting salary was only $1,000 less than her mother's!

Hospitals used to shy away from publishing definite salary figures when advertising for nurses. They resorted to euphemisms like "salary commensurate with experience and education." An empty phrase. Today's ads are much more specific.

An advertisement for a Washington, D.C., hospital says that RNs with 5 years of experience will start with an annual base salary of $36,310, while a new graduate will start with $28,459. (That's a 22% difference.) They also offer a 20% differential for permanent evenings and a 25% differential for permanent nights, along with "superpremium pay" for working additional shifts, guaranteed annual step increases, and *unlimited* salary progression.

That last phrase, "unlimited salary progression," is very significant. Traditionally, nurses have reached the top of the salary scales within 5 to 7 years. Some hospitals stretched that to 10 years. (You didn't make any more than the nurse who topped out in 7 years, it just took you longer to get there.) After you reached the top of the scale, only cost-of-living raises were given. Of course, those cost-of-living increases never actually matched increases in the cost of living. The end result was less and less buying power.

Fifteen years ago a new graduate started at an average salary of $16,000 and could expect to top out at $21,000, an increase of only 30% across the entire career lifespan. Slowly but surely, that percentage has inched upward from 35% in 1983 to 37% in 1985, 39% in 1987, 49% in 1991, and 51% in 1995.

How much is education worth? Only about 20% of hospitals pay registered nurses with baccalaureate degrees more than those with lesser education.

Perhaps you work for one of the few institutions that does reward educational efforts. Knowing your hospital pays more to nurses with degrees may be one of the reasons you are thinking of going back to college. You may even be among the thousands of nurses already working toward degrees. Did you ever stop to ask your hospital exactly how much your degree will be worth?

Looking at the guides to career opportunities published annually by nursing journals is quite an eye-opener. Hospitals throughout the United States spend big money on full-page advertisements hoping to entice nurses like you to come and work for them. In the 1992 guides they offered everything from free laundry service to Hawaiian vacations to $10,000 sign-on bonuses! Today most of those goodies are gone. Tomorrow, who knows?

Some hospitals still offer only a few cents more per hour for a BSN; some offer a few hundred more per year. One hospital offers a 3% differential for a BSN, another 3% for a master's, and also a 3% raise for certification. For a nurse making $40,000 per year, that would amount to an increase of just over $1,200 a year for a BSN ($41,200 to be exact). Add a master's or certification and it would amount to $42,400. It may be better than nothing but it's not much considering the time and money spent on education. That 1995 Earnings Survey in *RN* reported that "the influence education has on income appears to be negligible."

Of course, there are reasons other than financial gain to pursue higher education. Education often unlocks doors to job opportunities providing more personal and professional satisfaction.

Actually, the satisfactions of the nursing profession are seldom measured in terms of dollars or "sense." Nurses often defy logic by continuing to work in spite of physical strain, emotional drain, or lack of tangible rewards. An advertising executive has a plaque on her wall that reads:

> *In the ad game,*
> *the days are tough,*
> *the nights are long,*
> *and the work is emotionally demanding.*
> *But it's all worth it,*
> *because the rewards*
>   *are shallow,*
>   *transparent,*
> *and meaningless.*

In the nursing game the days are tough, the nights are long, and the work is emotionally demanding. But it's all worth it *because* of the rewards. Some of our rewards may be intangible, but they are far from being shallow, transparent, or meaningless.

If you have ever gotten misty-eyed reading first-person accounts in professional journals about "my most unforgettable patient," you know what I am talking about. We've all had unforgettable patients. And one special patient, vividly remembered, can carry a nurse through the frustrations of long hours, poor staffing, and bizarre scheduling.

Nursing is rich in intangible rewards. Have you ever thought about which intangibles are most important to you?

During an after-dinner conversation at an interdisciplinary conference, a doctor and a nurse discovered they had both been offered top positions at a major metropolitan hospital. Since the hospital was about to launch a highly specialized intensive care department, it was in search of the best medical and nursing professionals it could find.

As the two discussed their interviews, experiences, and observations, I listened intently. Both were struck by the magnitude of the project and intrigued by the challenge it promised. Both found the city appealing. Both mentioned the young, inexperienced staff that was in great need of guidance from seasoned professionals.

It was the hospital's great need that most impressed the nurse.

She was obviously struggling with her decision to accept or reject the hospital's offer.

Although the doctor also acknowledged the hospital's great need, he did not feel compelled to donate himself to their cause. He had already made his reply to the hospital's offer. He had declined.

Encouraging her to consider her own needs, not just the hospital's, the doctor said, "I know they will be extremely fortunate to get you. I just wonder if you will be equally fortunate to get them. Have you thought about what *you* will gain from this experience?"

The doctor went on to share his primary reason for declining the position. The hospital could not offer him what he valued most: first-rate peers. He had discovered the synergistic effect of working shoulder-to-shoulder with top-notch professionals. If he took the new position, he could give a lot to the young staff, but the kinds of things they could give him in return would not enhance his productivity. In his present position he enjoyed developing young staff, but he also enjoyed being surrounded by accomplished professionals who matched or exceeded his talent, intellect, curiosity, and drive.

How easy it is to forget our own needs when others' needs clamor for our attention! How difficult it is to maintain the proper balance between nourishing others and being nourished ourselves!

Striving to match our qualifications to the needs of the institution, we are often distracted from asking an equally important question: *do the institution's qualifications match our needs?*

Just how well are *your* needs being met by the institution for which you work? Considering everything from your present performance to your future prospects, how satisfied are you with your current job? Ask yourself the following questions:

1. Do I look forward to going to work each day?
2. Do I leave work feeling satisfied and successful?
3. What new skill or insight have I acquired this past week? Month? Year?
4. What old skill or knowledge have I mastered?
5. What one thing did I accomplish this week that will have lasting value?
6. What outstanding piece of nursing did I do this past week? Month? Year?
7. How am I using this job to meet my short-term goals? Long-term goals?

8. How will this job make me a better nurse?
9. Which of my fringe benefits do I consider most valuable?
10. Does my salary reflect my experience, education, and level of responsibility?
11. What are my opportunities for advancement in the next 12 months?
12. How would I describe the people I work with shoulder-to-shoulder each day? (Choose up to four words from the following list to describe them.)

WORD LIST	PEOPLE WORKING WITH ME
Informed	Nurses
Supportive	1. _____
Innovative	2. _____
Fair	3. _____
Creative	4. _____
Decisive	Doctors
Spirited	1. _____
Intelligent	2. _____
Caring	3. _____
Professional	4. _____
Trustworthy	Supervisors
Honest	1. _____
Reliable	2. _____
Organized	3. _____
Hard Working	4. _____
Humanitarian	Administrators
Efficient	1. _____
Effective	2. _____
Generous	3. _____
Skillful	4. _____
Enthusiastic	Other personnel
	1. _____
	2. _____
	3. _____
	4. _____

To survive in any job you need adequate amounts of:

FINANCIAL REWARD
INTELLECTUAL STIMULATION
EMOTIONAL SATISFACTION

To thrive, you need optimal amounts.

If you do not find your job financially rewarding, intellectually stimulating, and/or emotionally satisfying, it is time to find a new job. If you do not find the nursing profession financially rewarding, intellectually stimulating, and/or emotionally satisfying, it is time to find a new profession. *Or* it is time to do something to make your job and profession more "profitable" in the tangible and intangible ways you value most.

There's a word I like to borrow from economics. *Satisfice.* It's a combination of two words: *satisfy* and *sacrifice.* Satisfice is that point at which the satisfaction achieved justifies the sacrifices involved.

Sacrifice   **Satisfaction**

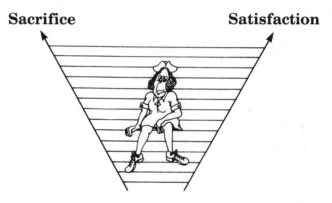

As you go onward and upward, you reach a level where you can live comfortably with the sacrifices and satisfactions life has to offer.

Great satisfaction usually involves great sacrifice. Ask any Olympic athlete or concert violinist. They sacrifice everything from careers to companionship in the single-minded pursuit of excellence.

Unfortunately, great sacrifice does not always ensure great satisfaction. You will find yourself in many ventures, jobs, and relationships that demand more from you than they are willing to give in return. A yard of sacrifice may only produce an inch of reward. You find yourself a victim of diminishing returns.

Sacrifice   **Satisfaction**

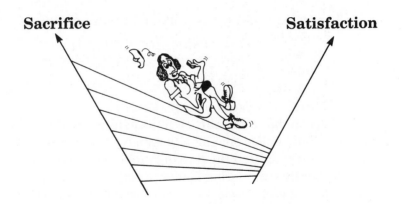

If the sacrifices greatly exceed the satisfactions, things can go downhill pretty fast.

Imagine for a moment that you have decided to be an Olympic-quality runner. Running becomes your life. It squeezes everything else out. It devours your time, energy, and money. You hire a coach, train constantly, buy special gear, and travel to competitions.

As a novice you don't expect to win right away, but you don't expect to lose consistently either. If you continue to trail behind, you may redouble your efforts. However, if your record still doesn't improve, you will probably be reluctant to invest any more time, energy, or money in the sport.

Eventually, discouraged by your lack of significant progress, you decide to cut your losses and run. Or rather, stop running. You either give it up altogether, or you become a recreational runner.

Years ago many of us dreamed of being Olympic-quality nurses. We trained hard and worked hard. We invested our time, energy, and money. Nursing became the center of our lives.

As novices we didn't expect big rewards or undue respect. We were willing to get additional coaching, training, and practice. Yet even after losing our amateur status, our profession was slow coming up with adequate rewards or recognition.

Thinking it was a personal problem and not a professional one, we redoubled our efforts. We got more education, took on new assignments, added responsibilities, switched into administration and education. Still the sacrifices demanded of us by our employers far exceeded our rewards.

Eventually, many of us decided to cut our losses and run. Nursing ceased to be the central focus of our lives. Some of us gave it up altogether. Others decided to become *Recreational Nurses*.

Recreational Nurses dabble in nursing. They no longer take their professional life too seriously. They like to keep a hand in nursing, but they have pulled their heads and hearts out. They work a day or two a week or donate time on the bloodmobile. Nursing provides a nice break from the other activities of their lives.

Rubber Nurses. Recreational Nurses. We are all RNs.

Sacrifice and satisfaction have tangible and intangible components. The tangible ones are more easily identified and calibrated. The intangible ones are highly individual.

The tangible rewards nursing offers may still need some adjustment, but the opportunity for intangible rewards is greater than in most jobs or professions. Those intangibles—sense of purpose, involvement, humanitarian goals—lift the satisfaction level enough to justify the sacrifices we must make to remain active in nursing.

Clinging to those intangibles can help save your professional life.

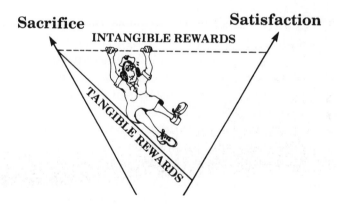

Saving your professional life may require shoring up both your tangible and intangible rewards. For example, if you are not satisfied with your salary, ask for a raise. It is surprising how few nurses ever do.

A sudden gust of courage propelled one nurse into her supervisor's office. She blurted out her request for a raise. The good news is she got it. The bad news is that it only amounted to 15 cents an hour.

If you want to be more successful than she was, first do your homework. Here are some tips that may help you:

Inventory your skills, knowledge, and abilities.
Estimate your contribution to the organization's goals.
Know whether you are seen as disposable or indispensable.
Know the precedents.
Envision all possible reactions to your request.
Anticipate questions that might be asked. Rehearse answers.
Make a formal appointment.
Have a specific dollar figure in mind.
Smile. Radiate confidence.
Focus on your worth, not on your need.

If your salary is tied to all other nurses' salaries, individual raises may be out. Collective bargaining takes over.

Regarding collective bargaining, all I can say is nurses need **help!** Nothing in our backgrounds has prepared us to negotiate intelligently and boldly. Hire experts. Heed their advice.

A midwestern director of nursing shared her disappointment with the outcome of recent negotiations at her hospital. As part of the management team, her attention and allegiance had to go to the greater goals of the organization. Yet she could not help feeling sad and frustrated as she watched the staff nurses settle for far less than the hospital was willing to offer.

Settling for less. Surviving but not thriving.

Nurses are the largest group of health care providers in the world. Many argue the only reason for hospitals to exist is to provide nursing care. Yet for decades JCAHO refused to recognize the importance of nursing and adamantly denied us a seat on the council. In 1992 they finally capitulated.

Perhaps they read the article in *U.S. News & World Report**that gave exclusive rankings of "America's Best Hospitals." In bold letters that article said, **"Nursing counts."** Their survey found, "The vast majority of doctors ranked quality of nursing care second, behind only the quality of the medical staff (physicians on the hospital payroll) as the chief predictor of capable hospital care—and ahead of state-of-the-art technology, research capabilities, and the quality of teaching in institutions affiliated with medical schools, all of which might seem to represent solid-gold indicators.

---

*Podlosky, Doug: America's best hospitals, *U.S. News & World Report* 112(23):63, June 15, 1992.

Apparently not. Indeed, geriatricians think the nursing staff is *the* most important factor."

The article goes on to give a miniprofile of the 43 top hospitals, listing the ratio of registered nurses to beds for each one. It might be interesting to compare how your hospital stacks up with these. Especially since a 1994 study by the University of Pennsylvania found that hospitals that employ more RNs relative to other nursing staff (aides, techs, LPNs) had a 5% lower mortality rate.

Nurses blew the whistle on San Francisco's Alta Vista Hospital, accusing it of misleading the public. Instead of being upfront and admitting that massive re-engineering, which resulted in the loss of many RN positions, was a cost-cutting activity, administration claimed it was a move to improve quality. They argued there would actually be more "caregivers." Well, as the University of Pennsylvania study points out, there are caregivers and then there are caregivers. RNs meant quality. RNs meant a lower mortality rate.

Of course, as hospitals reduce the number of beds, they also reduce the number of nurses needed. It's the *proportion* of nurses, relative to beds, that needs to be monitored. In California, for example, the RN share of the nursing workforce has dropped from 85% to 72%.

Getting rid of nurses may seem like a great way to save money. On the surface it is. For example, Milwaukee's Doyne Hospital calculated it could save $400,000 a year by replacing 14 RNs in its new outpatient clinic with nursing assistants. Physicians loudly protested. But to the bean counters, paying an aide $11/hour made more financial sense than paying an RN $20/hour.

It's just this kind of misuse and abuse of unlicensed staff that incensed Indiana Attorney General Pam Carter so much she set up an 800 number for people to report situations in which aides were taking on the duties of RNs and LPNs. In Cincinnati, nursing techs were found assessing patients, doing sterile procedures, inserting catheters, and giving complex wound care. The city council voted 7–1 to recommend that unlicensed techs be used only "in addition to an RN rather than replace the nurse."

This is supposed to be the Information Age. Intellectual assets are supposed to count. But today, in *every* industry, we see educated, experienced, competent, hard working, loyal workers being jettisoned and less educated, inexperienced, untested, cheap workers being brought on board.

For years nurses have been browbeaten into believing we are a liability, not an asset. Nurses don't drain the bottom line, we create the bottom line. Hospitals and nurses need each other. We need to work together on the problems facing health care. We need to look out for each other's interests.

You also need to look out for your own interests.

What will it take to satisfy you? Do you crave challenge, involvement, advancement, autonomy, support, first-class peers, flexible scheduling, new surroundings, better benefits, brighter prospects?

Everything is negotiable. You just have to decide what you want and what you are willing to sacrifice to get it. Ideally you won't have to sacrifice your profession.

Chapter 7

Prophet Sharing

Our satellite shows scattered hospices, frequent home births, and a possible increase in rehabilitation centers. Hospital per diem costs will reach highs of $800 and lows of $400. Gusts of old geezers are reported moving toward the southwest at speeds up to 55 mph. Film at eleven.

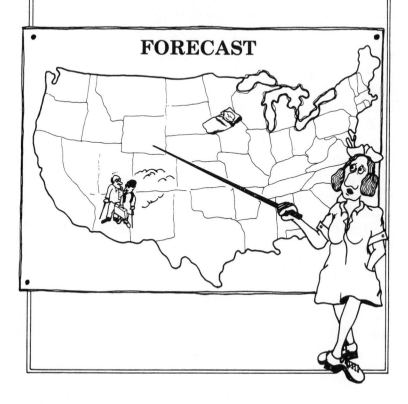

FORECAST

T HANKS for calling the Psychic Psych Nurse Hotline. How may I help you? No, don't tell me. You're worried about whether you'll have a job in the future. Right?"

"Right."

"Well, why do you think I started the Psychic Psych Nurse Hotline? I couldn't find any job in nursing that would pay me $4/minute. Do you know what that is an hour!?! And there's no more commuting, unless you count walking from the kitchen table to the phone. The best part is I have virtually no responsibility. I'm not accountable. No one can sue me for malpractice. That's what fine print is for. Look, there at the bottom of the screen where it says, 'Cost $4/minute. Must be a nursing school graduate or reasonable facsimile thereof. *For entertainment purposes only.* Dial 1-900-2SHRP4U.' Hey, would you sign up for my correspondence course and learn how to get rich by combining psychic powers with nursing process?"

In the future, nurses are going to have to live by their wits. This won't be easy because today's nurses are scared witless.

I don't know if there will be a job in your future. I do know there will be a lot of work to be done. The way that work is organized and compensated is what remains to be seen.

Health care seems to be undergoing some sort of seismic seizure. Like an earthquake, the ground keeps moving. No one is sure how things will shake out, how much structural damage will be done, or what the final costs will be. Just when things seem to be settling down, along comes an aftershock.

This "H.O.T." flyer was circulated at a nursing conference in Manitoba. Printed on fluorescent paper, it was impossible to ignore and its message was as alarming as the color of paper it was printed on.

This flyer is a jolting reminder of the unpredictable fortunes of nurses everywhere. One moment nurses are in great demand. The next moment nurses are on the unemployment line.

But we're not alone.

The cover on the September 25, 1995, issue of *Medical Economics* shows a stunned doctor holding a pink slip with the caption, "Will You Wind Up On the Unemployment Line?" The issue

---

H.O.T.
"HELPING OURSELVES TOGETHER"

♦ Are you unable to find a job?
♦ Have you been laid off?
♦ Have you been bumped?
♦ Are you anxious about workplace changes?

YOU ARE NOT ALONE

There are many nurses having similar experiences. If you would like to
share, with other nurses:

♦ Emotional Support
♦ Information
♦ Experiences
♦ Solutions

You are invited to drop in to the MARN Building anytime (647 Broadway
Avenue) between 7:30 and 9:30 p.m. on June 14th for a meeting.

ALL MEMBERS WELCOME!

---

ushered in a special three-part report on doctors' job prospects.

Health care professionals are finally experiencing what the
rest of the work world has been coping with for some time. Our job
security may have lasted longer than most other occupations and
professions, but now it's gone.

A nonpartisan private commission sponsored by the Pew Charitable Trusts of Philadelphia released predictions in November
1995 that by the year 2000 there will be as many as 150,000
excess doctors. They recommended that medical school graduates,
now running about 16,000 per year, be cut by 25% over the next 10

years. Furthermore, they recommended those reductions be achieved *not* by cutting class size but by *closing* some of the 127 medical schools in this country.

The commission also predicted *that hospital closings will throw as many as 300,000 nurses out of work.*

That's a middle-of-the-road estimate. Nursing leaders speculate that anywhere from 200,000 to 400,000 nursing positions in acute care will be lost by the turn of the century. Optimists suggest those nurses will be absorbed by home health and extended care facilities. But that transition, even if it occurs, will not be smooth or painless.

There may be an analogy with the closing of large, state-run psychiatric facilities a couple of decades ago. Those patients were supposed to be absorbed by community-based group homes and outpatient clinics. But the local facilities either never materialized or never developed sufficiently to handle the transfer. Many of those "set free" ended up homeless, sleeping on grates, and actively hallucinating while rummaging through the trash for their next meal.

While I don't expect nurses to end up sleeping on heating grates, I do think downsized nurses may be temporarily "homeless." There's a mismatch between the rate at which acute care is eliminating nursing positions and the rate at which alternate positions are opening. I haven't heard home health or extended care facilities yelling, "Yipee! Let's snap up all those surplus nurses!" They have budget constraints of their own. They're also being expected to do more with less. These agencies may not be as anxious to trade up as they are to dummy down.

Have you ever heard of aides for aides? An Illinois organization for extended care facilities invited me to speak at their annual meeting. Most of the participants were nursing managers and directors of nursing. Their focus was how to recruit and retain CNAs. They were desperate. They were also one of the most enthusiastic and creative groups of nurses I've ever worked with. At one point I asked them to share their best tip for either recruiting or retaining aides. They had wonderful examples:

- Giving a rose to the aide on her first day.
- Assigning an LPN to play "house mother" to new aides. She phones them the night before they report for duty and tells them she's looking forward to seeing them at 7 A.M. She nur-

tures, protects, and teaches them until they're ready to fly on their own.

♦ Giving them "play money" throughout the year for attendance, punctuality, mastering new skills, respecting residents, going above and beyond the call of duty. Then just before Christmas, they have an auction for prizes like TVs, weekend getaways, household items. The aides bid with the play money they've earned.

♦ Pizza parties . . . potlucks . . . root beer floats.

♦ Recognition day. CNA of the month, of the year.

♦ If they are working short of staff, they get an additional 75 cents an hour!

But the one that tickled me most was *giving the CNA an aide!* My mind started to wander. If a CNA has 6 weeks of training, how much training do you give a CNA's aide? Six hours? Six minutes? If they paid CNAs between $7–10/hour, how much would they pay a CNA's aide?

The nurse has been the workhorse in acute care. The aide has been the workhorse in extended care. Just because RNs are finding themselves displaced doesn't mean they will be replacing the CNAs.

Nurses in extended care or home health have routinely been paid less than their counterparts in acute care. And, if nurses glut the market, salaries could drop across the board.

Let's go back to that burning question: *Will there be a job in your future?*

There's only one way to make sure nurses stay off the unemployment line and continue to prosper. We have to create a public demand for professional nurses. We're going to have to market ourselves. We're going to have to advertise.

An excellent example of this is the American Nurses Association's pamphlet, "Every Patient Deserves a Nurse."

A hospital administrator, being interviewed on the radio about what downsizing would mean to patients, told the listeners not to worry. "We might lose some of the art but we won't lose any of the science."

Direct care givers, however, know the *art* of our craft is often more therapeutic than the science. Together they produce a synergistic effect. Patients know it too. The only people who don't seem to know it are the "bean counters."

Remember this little saying?

"Not everything that counts can be counted
and not everything that can be counted counts."

One advertising approach would be to call attention to the "countables." Anything we can put a numerical value on, especially those things that directly impact the bottom line. We may have a real *feel* for what nursing does but we often lack hard data, and bean counters aren't into feelings.

We need slogans. There are a couple of commercials running currently that I wish nursing could co-opt. One from Oldsmobile says, "It's your money. Demand better."

The public often loses sight of the fact that they are indeed paying for health care—through taxes, direct payments, and inflated price tags on all consumer goods. Health care is not a freebie. We need to remind them it's their money. We need to encourage them to demand better—to demand professional nursing care.

The other commercial, from the packing/shipping company Mailboxes Plus, says, "It's not *what* we do. It's *how* we do it." That's tailor made for nursing. Too bad we didn't think of it first.

Negative advertising may not be nice but it is very powerful. We could exploit tragedy and manipulate malpractice to our advantage. We could become *fearmongers*.

This is contrary to everything we've been taught, to everything we hold dear. But the hard truth is, fear sells. As headlines scream about the wrong foot being amputated, the wrong patient's respirator being disconnected, the wrong medication being given with fatal results, we could literally market nurses as "body guards."

Remember party invitations that said at the bottom B.Y.O.B., meaning bring your own booze? Well, I can envision a day when hospital admission forms will say B.Y.O.N.—Bring Your Own Nurse. A whole new breed of private duty nurses may rise to meet the demands of frightened, well-endowed patients.

No matter what happens, I am convinced nurses will be able to manage. The problem is nurses may not be able to lead.

According to the dictionary, *manage* means to direct, to control, to arrange, to supervise, to carry on, to get along. To *lead* means to guide, to play a principal role, to be ahead of, to aim in front of, to make the initial play, to show the way by going in advance.

The legacy of nursing is a legacy of management. Nurses have been shaped by society, by education, by our profession, and by the health care industry to manage. We've mastered management. No matter what circumstances we find ourselves in, we will carry on. Unfortunately, what we need now is the ability to lead.

Someone explained the difference between management and leadership this way. We're lost in the jungle. The manager climbs up a tree, looks around, and shouts out directions. The leader climbs up a tree, looks around, and shouts, "Wrong jungle!"

I think nurses have been in the wrong jungle for a long time. Being kicked out of acute care may be the best thing that ever happened to our profession. But the way nurses are kicking and screaming, you'd think we were being expelled from the Garden of Eden. Lighten up. Acute care was never paradise. It was always a jungle.

An operating room supervisor at a major university hospital was lamenting the fact they couldn't keep experienced OR nurses. It had become such a crisis they were forced to press new graduates into service even on complicated transplant cases.

I had never heard of such a thing. I told her I was very surprised. The turnover rate among OR nurses is extremely low. They love their jobs. Even during the nurse shortage, openings in the operating room were scarce. You had to wait for someone to retire or die.

She said they'd all been siphoned off by free-standing, outpatient surgical centers. Just about the time a new hire became competent, she was gone. The supervisor cited better hours, less work, more predictable caseloads, and no on-call time as reasons they jumped ship.

I told her I was still surprised. OR nurses take pride in their expertise. They love a challenge. They thrive on adrenalin and Mountain Dew. Frankly, their new jobs sounded kind of boring.

Then she dropped the other shoe, "Oh, yes, then there's the morale problem here . . ."

Those OR nurses liked the challenges of a university hospital setting but they weren't chumps. They could only take so much stress and abuse. Then one of the leaders climbed up a tree and shouted, "Wrong jungle!" Next thing you know, they were out of there.

Lots of nurses have decided they were in the wrong jungle. Some changed units, hospitals, clinical specialties; some moved into management, teaching, consulting, research; some went into clinics, industry, extended care, home health; some left nursing and health care behind.

The future of nursing is one thing. Your future may be another. If you don't like where health care is going, this may be an excellent time for you to break away.

Maybe it's time for you to leave your traditional practice setting and blaze a new trail. Like the nurse in Boston who bought a small hotel and opened a bed and breakfast for new moms and dads. They check out of the hospital and into her B & B. For $125 a night they can stay as long as they like. Instead of maid service they have nursing service. The new parents can learn how to feed, bathe, and generally cope with their bundle of joy while getting the rest, reassurance, and support they need.

Or the nurse in Vienna, Virginia, who opened her own home for elder care 8 years ago. She told me she can accomodate three or four. One is a 91-year-old man who's been with her 6 years and "is still going strong." She employs a home health aide during the week and an LPN on weekends or whenever she needs to be gone. She didn't give me specifics but she did say it was "very profitable." Perhaps instead of "nursing homes" we may see more "nurse's homes" open for business in the future.

To lead, nurses not only have to seize opportunities, we have to create them. We have to figure out what our customers want.

In his thought provoking book *Managing the Future: 10 Driving Forces of Change for the '90s* (G.P. Putnam's Sons, 1991), Robert B. Tucker says there are 10 things businesses must address if they are to stay viable:

1. Speed
2. Convenience
3. Age Waves
4. Choice
5. Lifestyle
6. Discounting
7. Value-Adding
8. Customer Service
9. Techno-Edge
10. Quality

He explains that a "driving force" is stronger and longer lasting than a trend or a fad. Future success depends on the ability to meet both internal and external customers' needs in relationship to these forces.

Use those 10 simple words to brainstorm ways to improve nursing's products and services. Ask yourself: How can we make things faster, cheaper, more valuable, more convenient? How can we better accomodate the young, the old, the rural, the urban, the affluent, the poor? How can we stay on the cutting edge? How can we improve customer service? How can we guarantee quality?

"Attention K-Mart Shoppers! Under the flashing blue light in the center aisle you will find our nurse. For the next 5 minutes only, physical assessments half price."

That example combines several of the driving forces—speed, convenience, lifestyle, discounting, *and* customer service.

A fantasy of the future? Not really. Health care clinics have already been established in many shopping malls. Some even provide patients with beepers to carry while they're shopping. Then, when the doctor is ready to see them, their beeper sounds, and they return for their appointment.

As competition for patients increases, expect to see more creative ventures. Hospitals are already offering everything from steak and champagne to money-back guarantees in hopes of luring patients. Everyone is scrambling for the vanishing health care dollar.

Collectively, we have all been screaming for lower health care costs. Individually, however, we still believe that when it comes to our *own* care, "Money is no object!"

But money is an object. You don't have to be much of a prophet to predict a future based on profit. Competition is already fierce. "For-profit" hospitals are siphoning off the well-endowed, well-insured patients, leaving the "not-for-profit" hospitals with the indigent, uninsured patients. While one hospital grabs all the profitable obstetrical business, another corners the market on coronary care. A bonanza for one hospital may mean bankruptcy for another.

That may not be the way it *should* be. That's the way it *is*.

If you want to see nursing in the future and your future in nursing, open your eyes. The first thing you will see is a computer. When you think of computers, do you smile or grimace? If you smile, you're ready for the future. If you grimace, you're in trouble.

Just for starters, computers hold the key to simplifying and reducing paperwork. One group of nurses was won over completely when their system computerized doctors' orders. Each doctor was required to enter orders, wait for the print-out, make necessary corrections, and then hand them over to the nurse. Nurses no longer had to try to decipher illegible handwriting, struggle to read minds, or waste time tracking down doctors for clarification. They quickly concluded that computers are a nurse's best friend.

Some nurses already telecommute to work. A drug company hired one to track dozens of patients throughout the United States who were on the same treatment protocol. She said, "I've never seen their faces but I talk to them via computer every day. They've become like family." Patients in remote geographic areas already "log on" to talk to their nurses. In 1993 John Thomas of Arlington, Virginia, developed the CURE Network. He and his 50 volunteers salvage old computers and train mentally ill people to become computer literate. The nonprofit group is creating a local electronic bulletin board geared to disabled and homebound people. No matter what disease you have, if you have a computer, you can get instant access to information and support groups.

Nursing organizations are going on-line. Nancy Sharp, Executive Director of the American College of Nurse Practitioners in Washington, D.C., told me her goal is to take all 49,500 nurse practitioners into cyberspace. She wants them electronically linked.

In addition to being computerized, here's what some nurses predict nursing's future to be:

"Providing quantity of life without quality"
"Return to acute care"
"Teaching, planning, coordinating"
"*Intense* intensive care!"
"Independent, stressful, specialized"
"Management from afar—less actual patient involvement"
"Increasingly community-oriented"
"More home health"
"More technical, less personal"
"Fanatic cost containment!"

Obviously nurses don't look too far into the future. Most of the items on this list were implemented yesterday.

Getting nurses to concentrate on the future isn't easy. We're too busy just getting through *today*. And, if tomorrow is anything like today, we'd rather not think about it at all.

Nurses tend to fight the future. We insist on swimming upstream. We complain, "The river shouldn't be running this way. It ought to run in the other direction."

Under great protest we are swept along. We cling to traditions, like rocks in a fast-moving stream, until the current overpowers us. We arrive in the future battered, bruised, exhausted . . . and late.

If we could learn to let go of the past and swim with the current, we might arrive in the future healthy, wealthy, wise . . . and on time.

Here are some of the things nurses say they would like to see in their future:

"More control over the work situation"
"Better quality of life for patients"
"Promotion of wellness, independence, and self-care"
"Fewer 'housekeeping' tasks for nurses"
"Autonomy is a must!"
"Treating and educating patients as whole beings"
"Emphasis on prevention"
"Third-party payment"
"Salaries commensurate with expertise"
"Affordable, accessible health care"

When asked what they are doing to bring these things into being, they fall silent. Nurses need to learn that if they want to influence the future, they have to go where the future is being influenced.

For example, have you ever attended the board meeting at your hospital? Few nurses have. They are too busy giving bedbaths to bother with such stuff and nonsense. Unfortunately, while you're at the bedside, your future is being determined in the boardroom.

Every day, hundreds or thousands of miles away in your state or national capital, politicians are making decisions and establishing policies that will directly influence your ability to give high-quality care at the bedside. Yet when was the last time you wrote to a member of Congress, gave testimony at a hearing, or marched up the capitol steps in protest? Think about it.

As I said, one way for nurses and nursing to stay viable is to figure out what consumers will want and need in the future. A good starting point is to examine the products and services available today. Which ones are lacking in quality or quantity?

What do health care consumers want? Exasperated nurses moan that patients want everything from "mind reading" to "maid service." Patients want "150% of my time and attention." Patients say, "Fix me—but I don't want to have to do anything to help myself." Another writes, "Champagne on a beer budget."

Today's patients are impatient. They want speed and convenience. Free-standing, immediate care centers have sprung up all over the landscape to service people who have no time to wait.

Two nurse practitioners in Washington state opened their own clinic. In their market survey they discovered people were less concerned about price and whether a doctor or a nurse provided care; their prime concern was convenience. Those nurse practitioners effectively set up a one-stop health-care shop by leasing space to a dentist and a pharmacist and providing expanded hours to meet customers' needs.

Responding to the needs of dual-career families, a pediatric clinic in my neighborhood is open only from 6 P.M. to midnight. It is a perfect solution for working parents who find it difficult, if not impossible, to keep daytime appointments.

Some nurses see the burgeoning elderly population as a problem. Others see it as an opportunity. Workshop groups have lively discussions about future business opportunities for nursing in areas like elderly day care, intermediate care (between hospital and home or nursing home), in-the-home nursing, educational programs aimed at the elderly, and preventive health packages, including nutritional and social programs.

Nurses think health care consumers lack information both in quantity and quality. They see a need for:

"Adequate information on drugs and their use"
"Honest advertising"
"Interpreters of medical jargon"
"Truly informed consent"
"Better teaching concerning diagnosis, treatment alternatives, lifestyle adjustments"
"Adequate, accurate explanations of invasive procedures"
"Understandable information"

"More health maintenance information"
"Information on the credibility of doctors—which are really the
    best?"
"Better hospital orientation, clearer information, more choice"
"Knowledge of medications in layperson's terms"
"Diet *how's* and *why's*"
"Information on prices"
"Better understanding of where a health care dollar goes"
"Awareness of extent to which doctors regulate and control the
    system"
"Facts!"

Does this list suggest any future opportunities to you? If not,
try the next list. It centers on providing "quality" service. Nurses
feel health care consumers have a desire or need for:

"Better-quality emergency room care"
"Privacy, self-respect, dignity"
"Personalized attention"
"Caring! Treatment as human beings"
"Discharge planning that provides enough support for wellness
    instead of just meeting the needs of illness"
"More time"
"Psychological support"
"Counseling"
"Access to modern techniques and knowledge"
"Respect for their time—less waiting!"
"Sense of continuity"
"Mutual respect between client and provider"
"Care planned to meet their needs, not the doctor's needs"
"Protection of patient's rights
"Give choices"
"Listen!"
"Understanding . . . compassion . . . comfort . . . security"
"Top priority"
"Hospice"
"Involvement in decision making"
"Optimal care"
"The right to sexual activity in an acute care setting"
"Attention!"

If nurses can provide "quality care with no frills and low bills," our future seems assured.

Nursing employment opportunities may fluctuate and cycle just as they do in most other occupations. Feast or famine? In either event your professional future depends on your ability to find the best job possible. If it's a matter of survival, any job may be the right job. If you're more concerned with "thrival," you will have to be more creative and ingenious than ever before.

Take Jane for example. She hated her job. Even though she knew the job market for nurses was tight, she decided to risk everything. First, she stockpiled 3 months' salary. Then she quit. The job search she had carefully planned would be a full-time effort.

She began visiting local hospitals, spending time just sitting in the lobby, riding the elevators, eating in the cafeterias, chatting with visitors and personnel, reading in-house publications, studying bulletin boards, walking through the units. When she decided a hospital would be a good place to work, she asked for the name of the head nurse in her preferred specialty.

Then she would put on her best suit, go to the unit, and introduce herself. Jane would tell the head nurse she realized she was busy right now but would ask for an appointment to discuss career opportunities at a later date. Not one head nurse refused.

During these informational interviews, Jane learned a great deal more about the hospital, the unit, the nurse manager, the daily routine, and the employment possibilities. She would leave a copy of her resume. Afterward, she wrote each head nurse a thank-you note.

Next Jane would go to personnel and inquire about any current openings for nurses. She filled out job application forms.

Every week she would make the rounds of the personnel departments to see if any new jobs had been posted. She would say hello and remind them she was still actively looking. Then, every 7 to 10 days, she would pop up on the unit. She'd smile, say hi, and tell the head nurse she'd just been down in personnel and was still hoping for something to open up.

To Jane's surprise she was offered three management positions, even though she had no management experience whatsoever! While she was flattered, that was not the type of job she wanted. She held out. In less than 2 months, she was offered her ideal job. She's never been happier.

In the best of times or the worst of times, a job-hunting nurse needs a sound résumé. That résumé should include:

Name, address, and phone number
Educational experience
Work experience
Special skills or certifications
States in which licensed
Professional organizations

The résumé should be concise, clear, clean, complete, and kept to a single page. Some nurses find it difficult to confine their résumé to one page, whereas others complain theirs would fit on a postage stamp. If your career is lengthy and varied, select highlights and offer more details on request. If your résumé is too thin, expand on job titles by including descriptions of activities or duties performed. You might also add personal interests or continuing education seminars attended to round out a full page.

When constructing your résumé, maximize your assets. Don't overlook them. Take credit for your achievements. Use only positive words and phrases. Make use of action verbs like *improved, implemented, directed, administered, supervised, taught, prepared, conducted, established, planned,* and *evaluated.*

Do not list references on your résumé. Offer them upon request after you are sure there is mutual interest between you and the prospective employer.

A cover letter should accompany your résumé. Although the résumé remains constant, the cover letter is personalized for each situation. It might include how you found out about the opening, why you are interested in the position, and the skills and qualities you possess that make you well suited to their needs. The tone should be confident and enthusiastic, so the recruiter or director will be enticed into granting an interview.

When preparing for the interview, find out everything possible about the position, the institution, and the person conducting the interview.

Ask yourself if you are just looking for work (survival) or trying to make a career-connected move (thrival).

Rehearse responses to possible questions. Why do you want to change jobs? What were your duties in your last job? Why do you want this particular job? What is your nursing philosophy? And the ever-popular, "Tell me about youself."

Make a list of concrete examples demonstrating your ability to work efficiently and effectively. Concentrate on your strengths. Practice wording everything, including your shortcomings, in a positive manner.

Carry a notepad and pen with you. Bring along a list of questions you will want answered before making a decision. Take an extra copy of your résumé and a list of three professional references including name, title, address, and phone number.

Dress in a conservative, professional manner. Don't smoke or chew gum.

Arrive on time or just moments before the scheduled appointment. Smile. Walk tall. Speak in a well-modulated voice. Maintain eye contact. Be friendly, respectful, and attentive. Exude confidence.

To decrease your nervousness during the interview try remembering this is a two-way street. Yes, they are interviewing you, but you are also interviewing them.

If at all possible visit the institution a few days before the interview and take a long, leisurely look around. Survey the grounds. Spend time eavesdropping in the cafeteria. Ask directions from different staff members. You can quickly assess whether this is an institution where people thrive or fight to survive.

Make your own observations. How confident, enthusiastic, and professional is the person conducting the interview? How well prepared is she? Is she evasive? Vague? Authoritarian? Would you like to work with or for this person?

Let the interviewer guide the session. Answer questions honestly and candidly. If a question takes you by surprise, don't feel compelled to blurt out an answer. Tell the interviewer you would like to give it some thought. Ask permission to come back to that question later.

When your turn comes to ask questions, consult your list. Inquire about patient care assignments, philosophies, staffing policies, continuing education opportunities, and advancement possibilities. Finally, if the information hasn't been offered, ask about salary, scheduling or shift requirements, and fringe benefits.

At the close of the interview, summarize your intent, interests, and hopes. If you are definitely not interested in the position, say so as tactfully as possible. If you are very interested, convey that message clearly. Negotiate a definite time frame in which they will let you know about the position or you will let them know about your decision.

If they offer you the job right on the spot, chances are they are desperate. If you accept right on the spot, you are desperate. Take your time, or you may be taken.

Follow up the interview with a brief thank-you note. Even if this position doesn't work out, there may be attractive future openings coming up. Your note will help them remember you as a very professional person with a lot of potential.

Are you prepared for future employment in nursing? Do you know where the jobs will most likely be? Predicted boom areas include hospice units and hospital-based in-home services. Other areas expected to grow rapidly include rehabilitation, oncology, IV therapy, orthopedics, and ambulatory units.

The larger the hospital, the more likely a BSN degree will be required in the near future. Nurses with special certification will also be in demand. Openings for "generic" nurses may decrease as demand for specialized nurses increases.

When Abbott Northwestern Hospital opened a highly specialized cardiovascular stepdown unit, the decision was made to require that applicants have a bachelor's degree. Since the nurse shortage was quite a problem at the time, some worried they would not get enough qualified candidates. They received 300 applicants for the 17 positions! The competition was fierce. Nurses want to work where knowledge and competence are valued.

Is there a promotion in your future? That will probably depend on your willingness to obtain a degree and get special certification. Hard work is rarely the key to a promotion. The key is visibility—having the people at the top recognize you and your ability.

In first-rate institutions promotions go to those who are self-motivated, confident, eager, and ambitious. In second-rate institutions promotions go to those who are long-suffering, submissive, and compliant. First-rate institutions are more concerned with results. Second-rate ones focus on efforts. To determine which kind of institution you are in, look up the organizational ladder at least two or three rungs.

Remember, your professional environment can change overnight. That's what happened to Angela. Her supervisor, a grand champion for nurses and nursing, was recruited for a top position at a hospital far away. Suddenly Angela found herself reporting to a former peer who could best be described as a wimp.

Angela was a clinical nurse specialist on a neonatal unit tyrannized by a medical director who distained women in general and nurses in particular. The two frequently locked horns. While he did not like her, he grudgingly respected her professional expertise.

Knowing the new supervisor was a peace-at-any-price pushover, the doctor began to strut and bluster. He made demands. She acquiesced. He made demands of Angela. She held her ground. He complained to the supervisor. Angela was called in and *ordered* to capitulate without any discussion of what was professionally appropriate. The parting shot was a thinly veiled threat that Angela "should just be happy to have a job."

That was the day Angela updated her résumé. She sent out three. The results were immediate. *Six* interviews and two job offers.

Angela credits her network. When she had arrived in that job and that city three years earlier, she had phoned or written every other neonatal clinical nurse specialist in the area to introduce herself. They had formed a very active professional network. The moment word got out that Angela was "on the move," the network kicked in. Her résumé was passed from hand to hand, from one organization to another. She was quickly snapped up.

When she tendered her resignation, the supervisor was shocked, but the medical director was stunned. He begged her to stay. He told her they could work things out. He urged her to think of what was best for the unit.

Angela calmly told him it was not negotiable. She was gone.

A lesser person would probably gloat, but Angela shares this with me in a very low-key, matter-of-fact manner. She is a professional. She doesn't whine, pout, fret, hold grudges, or waste time wondering about what might have been. Angela doesn't make threats, she makes decisions.

Frankly, she doesn't understand nurses who stay in jobs that make them miserable. Life is too short. There's too much to be done.

The job Angela took might surprise you. As I write this she's being oriented as an emergency room staff nurse. She laughs when she talks about going from "expert" to "stupid" in just one day. The transition is tough, but it has its upside. As a clinical nurse specialist, she put in close to 60 hours a week. As a staff nurse she works 40, and because of shift differentials, is actually paid more! The nicest bonus is having time for a personal life again.

Her new job is part of a bigger plan. Angela is on her way to becoming a family nurse practitioner. One of the school's requirements is two years of caring for adult patients. Hence the job in the ER. Although she loves the "wee ones," she thinks this credential will make her more marketable. By reinventing herself, Angela is securing her place in the future.

When good jobs are so hard to find, you may have to go out and create one. Today, more than ever before, nurses are being forced to get their act together and take it on the road. Here is one nurse's success story:

> One year ago on a dark and black Friday afternoon in April, my position, along with four of my colleagues', was suddenly dissolved. Wiped out of existence! Kaputt! We were all given until September to either find new positions in our institution or obtain positions elsewhere.
>
> Well, after the shock and tears were over, determination set in. I decided I was good for my institution and I could make a place for myself. I was going to help my institution in spite of itself!
>
> Gaining the support of one of my displaced colleagues, I began to tackle the problem. For a long time it had been my premise that our education department could support its in-house activities by marketing its resources to outside institutions.
>
> First, I did the necessary field research. I visited outlying agencies and assessed their needs. I took a couple of business courses, including one specifically geared to health care marketing. Then I wrote a marketing proposal (the first ever written at our "sophisticated" institution).
>
> My colleague and I presented our proposal to the administrator. *It was approved and funded as a pilot project!!!*
>
> Our pilot project lasted 6 months. I evaluated the data then revised the marketing objectives and plans. I presented the evaluation to the administrator myself. Again I passed inspection and the project was continued. Success!
>
> If the project flops tomorrow, it doesn't matter. I have learned so much. It was scary at times and loads of work. But I made many new contacts, mastered moving things through red tape, and learned whom to work with and whom to work around.
>
> This experience, which began as a horrible problem (complete with

tears), ended as my greatest career opportunity. If my old job hadn't been "dissolved," I would have missed a lot of fun, excitement, and stimulation. I would never have become the knowledgeable, confident professional I am today.

Whether you like it or not, the future arrives daily. You can resist it, or you can run forward to meet it. The way the future is approached is what separates nurses who survive from those who thrive.

Welcome to the future!

Chapter 8

Procrastination

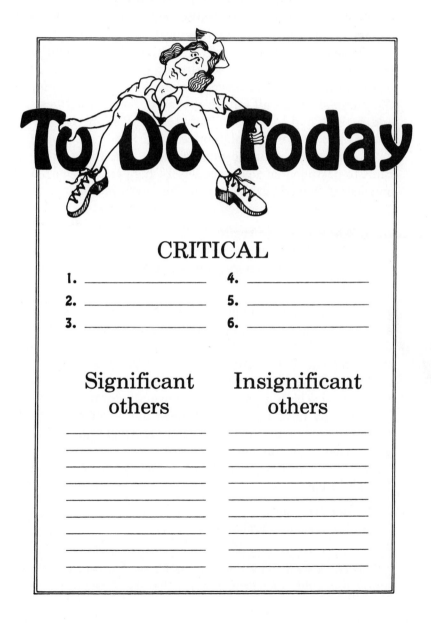

CRITICAL

1. _____   4. _____
2. _____   5. _____
3. _____   6. _____

Significant others	Insignificant others
_____	_____
_____	_____
_____	_____
_____	_____
_____	_____
_____	_____
_____	_____

W HILE developing the third edition of *STAT: Special Techniques in Assertiveness Training for Women in the Health Professions,** I expanded the annotated bibliography. Reviewing one of the new additions titled "Overcoming Procrastination," I facetiously wrote, "I haven't gotten around to reading this one yet."

It was true. I owned the book for 3 years before I finally read it. Like many people I am an inveterate procrastinator.

For example, when I began writing the first edition of this book, the nurse shortage was already excruciating and seemed to be escalating daily. As I dawdled along, the economy collapsed, and the nurse shortage all but disappeared. Some of my best rantings and ravings had to be reevaluated and, alas, rewritten. Procrastination often demands a high price.

To procrastinate is to put off doing something until a future time, to postpone or delay needlessly. It's perfectly normal. Everyone does it. Nobody *wants* to do it, but everyone does it.

The three most common reasons for procrastination are:

1. Not wanting to begin.
2. Not knowing where to begin.
3. Not knowing where to begin, even if you wanted to begin, which you don't.

What have you been putting off or needlessly delaying? Getting a physical examination, making a dental appointment, starting a diet, knitting a sweater, looking for a job, disciplining an employee, obtaining a divorce, writing an article, attending college?

Some of the above tasks are unpleasant. Some are overwhelming. Some are both unpleasant and overwhelming.

You may have lots of good ideas and even more good intentions, but somehow time keeps slipping away and you never quite get started . . . or finished.

Self-help books will tell you to follow something like these "simple" steps:

1. Set priorities.
2. Focus on one problem at a time.

---

*Chenevert, Melodie: *STAT: Special techniques in assertiveness training for women in the health professions,* ed. 3, St. Louis, 1988, Mosby.

3. Give yourself a deadline and stick to it.
4. Don't sidestep difficult problems.
5. Remember, only God is perfect.

Seems simple enough, doesn't it? What those self-help books fail to tell you is that you may require years of psychotherapy to accomplish any one of the above.

Take the first directive: set priorities. When you set priorities, you are required to make decisions. Not only do you have to decide what you are going to do, you have to decide what you are *not going* to do.

Women often lack the self-confidence to be decisive. Fearful of making the "wrong" decision, we hesitate to make any decision. We overlook the fact that not to decide is to decide. It is decision by default. If you delay a decision long enough, it will be made for you. "This offer expires at midnight."

We tend to see choices as right or wrong, black or white, all or nothing. Although some choices may prove better than others, few involve such extremes. However, all decisions do involve an element of risk, and unfortunately, women view risk as entirely negative. Women avoid risk. Women avoid making decisions.

The next time you are faced with an important choice, try viewing it as an *opportunity* instead of a problem. Most of us seize opportunities. All of us avoid problems.

Procrastinators typically spend more time and energy inventing excuses than it would take to invent solutions. Do any of these sound familiar?

"I'm just not in a creative mood."
"I'll start first thing tomorrow."
"Because of circumstances beyond my control. . . ."
"If I can't do it right, I won't do it at all."
"Not tonight. I have a headache."
"As soon as I solve my other problems, I'll get right on it."
"All work and no play. . . ."
"I work better under pressure."

Exploring the root causes of your procrastination may be a fascinating pastime, but it won't solve the problem. Insight doesn't solve problems, *action* does.

Five-Minute Antidote for Inertia

Time-management experts recognize that the biggest hurdle to overcome is inertia. The old saying about the longest journey beginning with a single step is the basis for the 5-minute plan. Here is a practically painless way to take the first step.

Strike a bargain with yourself. Agree to give some miserable task 5 minutes of your time. That's right—just 5 minutes. You can stand almost anything for that length of time.

Set a timer and begin. When the timer rings, you may quit. That's fine. You have kept your bargain.

Instead of quitting immediately, you may decide to work just 5 minutes more. Reset the timer and continue.

Once you are in motion, you may find it hard to stop. The activity builds a momentum that will probably carry you far beyond those first 5 minutes. It is not only possible, it's highly probable that you won't even *want* to stop.

This gimmick is rather like setting your wristwatch 5 minutes fast to keep from being late. It's deceptively simple, but it works.

When I did a workshop for Walter Reed Army Medical Center, a colonel in the audience told me she had read this tip in the *Pro-Nurse Handbook* and for 2 years she had on her to-do list "Buy a kitchen timer." About 6 months before the workshop she had purchased one. She agreed it was a good idea and then she told me of another way she uses the timer. Now I use her method.

Every day she makes two lists side by side on the same sheet of paper. One is her "have-to-do" list and beside it is her "want-to-do" list. She takes her timer and sets it for 60 minutes. She works on her have-to-do's. When it rings she resets the timer and shifts to her want-to-do's. She said her productivity went right through the roof. It is a great idea. Try it. It works.

Listless?

For those who just don't seem to know where to begin, making a "TO DO" list is helpful. A fresh list should be made each day.

If you generate too lengthy a list, you may be so overwhelmed all you can do is take two aspirin and a nap. Limit the list to the six most important things you have to accomplish. Set priorities on them. It doesn't matter whether you split your list into sections as the cartoon at the beginning of this chapter does, use a star system, or color-code the list with red, green, and blue ink. Start with the most important item and work it through to a conclusion. Then go on to number two.

If the same item shows up on your list day after day, you have a problem. You are procrastinating. Make the decision to *Do It Now* or cross it off your list. Either way you will be more productive.

CAUTION: Sometimes making a list gives you a false sense of accomplishment. A list is a plan, not a product.

One of the reasons procrastinators need a list is because we honestly do not remember from one moment to the next what our goals are. If we do not have them written down for constant reference, we forget.

We are easily distracted. We are the kind of people who can walk by the TV set and the next thing you know 2 hours of life have vanished. They are gone forever. Or perhaps you are finally going to write that article for professional publication. On your way to the typewriter, you pass by the laundry hamper. You decide to toss in a load of clothes. There is no reason they can't be washing while you are writing. Then you notice you are running low on detergent. You think, "I should dash to the store. While I'm at it, I should pick up something for dinner."

The next thing you know it is 6 months later. And you have not written one paragraph on that article for publication.

Every couple of weeks review your lists to see if you are accomplishing anything of permanent value. It is easy to be so swamped with day-to-day activities that no constructive action is being taken toward some of your long-range goals. Remember, they are only goals if you are working toward them. Otherwise, they are merely dreams. Procrastinators are dreamers.

Do It Now!

Procrastinators have the habit of putting everything off until "later." To kick the habit, take action. *Do It Now!*

Put this book down! Get up and make that phone call, pay that bill, write that letter, clean that oven, enroll in that class, do those push-ups!

You may be a person haunted by a half-knitted afghan at the back of your closet. Everytime you handle it, you feel a sense of failure. "I *should* finish this afghan. I've been moving it around for 15 years." Give that almost-heirloom to a relative or donate it to Goodwill Industries. Get it out of your closet and into someone else's. You'll feel terrific.

Whenever possible take care of things that cross your desk (or your mind) right on the spot. If you don't, a stack of "stuff" will sprout and quickly engulf your desk, mantel, or dining-room table. This stack usually consists of unanswered letters, bills, announcements, appeals, special offers, coupons, newspapers, magazines, receipts, and recipes.

Strive to handle each piece of paper only once. As you sort the daily mail, be decisive. Do you really want to subscribe to this magazine? Do you really want to contribute to this charity? Do you really want to read last Sunday's newspaper? If the answer to these questions is yes, *Do It Now*. If the answer is maybe, trash it. Adopt the motto "If in doubt, throw it out!"

For those of you who are pack rats and cannot bring yourself to throw papers away, this is the next best piece of advice I ever heard. Everytime you handle that paper, tear part of it off. Pretty soon it self-destructs.

When you have an unpleasant task to perform, such as disciplining an employee, it is natural to want to avoid the task altogether. Accept the fact that some things are absolutely unavoidable. The longer you delay, the more you worry. As your anxiety increases, your ability to concentrate decreases. Your efficiency and effectiveness plummet.

Writing in *Getting Things Done: The ABC's of Time Management,** Edwin C. Bliss recommends starting each day by doing the most unpleasant thing on your "TO DO" list. Getting that thing out of the way first will make you feel exhilarated, almost euphoric. According to the author, an effective person approaches

---

*Bliss, Edwin C.: *Getting things done: The ABC's of time management*, New York, 1991, Charles Scribner's Sons.

unpleasant tasks by saying, "This task is unpleasant, but it must be done; therefore I will do it now so I can forget about it."

Go to Pieces

Because I love quilts so much, I used to wonder if I had the talent and perseverance to make one. Luckily, someone had invented a quilt-as-you-go method that allowed me to complete one little 12-inch block at a time. The grand plan was to finish 20 or 30 blocks and join them together to make a quilt.

Before I actually tried my hand at quilting, I aspired to making a queen-sized quilt. After struggling a few hours, I revised my goals and began thinking about a crib-sized quilt. I ended up making a pillow. One block was all I managed to complete.

I learned some valuable lessons from that experience: (1) you never know what you can (or can't) do until you actually try; (2) quilts can be bought; and (3) the key to accomplishing any large task is to break it down into little pieces. This applies to making a quilt, learning a new language, painting the house, cleaning the attic, writing a book, moving across country, or getting a college education.

College degrees, like quilts, can be pretty and practical or pretty impractical. It all depends on how they are made and how they are used.

If you are one of the many nurses who has been thinking about returning to school but are not sure you have the talent or perseverance required, try the learn-as-you-go method. Instead of letting the magnitude of the project overwhelm you, find a manageable piece.

Talk with a college advisor and have her spell out exactly what the college will require of you. Then take the college catalogue and read the course descriptions. Choose a course that not only meets college requirements but meets your personal requirements as well.

Choosing *one* class that looks interesting and has practical application in your real world will give you a sample of what it is like to be back in school. If you choose wisely, the class will be a satisfying experience in itself and also double as the first step toward a degree.

Committing yourself to a few weeks of classwork is less intimidating than committing to years of schooling. At any time you can revise your goals. After all, they are *your* goals.

On completing the first class, you may opt to take another, thus inching toward a degree. You may zealously decide to enroll full time. On the other hand, you may discover you do not want to be a student now or ever again. Working on your bachelor's degree can be crossed off your "TO DO" list. Redirect that time, energy, talent, and money toward something you really do want to do.

Time and Punishment

Behaviorists say that any activity followed by a reward is remembered pleasantly and tends to be repeated. Therefore, if you reward yourself for performing promptly, you will be on your way to breaking the procrastination habit.

Rewards may involve food, fun, friendship, or anything else you enjoy and usually indulge in each day. If you have a passion for coffee, you might decide to withhold coffee until you finish some appointed task. You allow yourself a cup of coffee only *after* you clean the closet, write Aunt Harriet, or finish your income tax forms. Until you complete your task, there will be no television, no phone calls, no luncheons, no shopping, or no bubble bath.

Some extremely stubborn procrastinators find the reward system needs to be enhanced by a punishment system. For example, if you fail to meet your deadline, you not only lose the reward, you enforce a punishment. You make yourself do something you hate—walk to work, take a cold shower, eat artichokes for breakfast, donate money to a political cause you oppose, or take a person you dislike to lunch.

Fear of Trying

There are many reasons why women may be more prone to procrastination than men. Little boys are encouraged to approach life in a rough-and-tumble manner. They are encouraged to "go for it!"

Sure boys get hurt. That's part of life. But that's not supposed to be part of life for little girls.

Girls are cautioned to approach life in a safety-first manner. Just the thought of getting hurt is enough to deter girls from doing anything potentially dangerous. Unfortunately, anything potentially dangerous is also potentially fun and profitable.

Instead of wholeheartedly participating in life's scramble, girls sit on the sidelines. They grow up to be ladies-in-waiting, women who are not action-oriented but reaction-oriented. Programmed to observe events and accept decisions, they pride themselves on their ability to respond, compromise, and accommodate.

The saying "If life hands you a lemon, make lemonade" is descriptive of the way women are expected to handle life. Wait and see what life hands you, then do the best you can.

Goals can cause conflict for women because we have traditionally molded our lives around the goals of others. Once on the trail of our own goals, we are no longer as available as we once were. We are no longer as flexible. We can no longer be found cheering on the sidelines.

Sometimes that causes problems for other people, such as our husbands, children, parents, pastors, and employers. Since their problems have always been our problems, they may pressure us to postpone our own goals.

When you are feeling pressured, remember what management expert Peter F. Drucker says, "Most executives have learned that what one postpones, one actually abandons."

Don't postpone or abandon your goals. Risk going after what you want. Don't wait for life to hand you a lemon, go out and pick what you really want.

If you just take life as it happens, you can always blame your misfortunes on luck or fate. Although that may dilute failure, it also waters down success because you can't take credit for your good fortune either.

Procrastinators are great believers in luck and fate.

Productive people have learned that future gain usually requires present pain. They have learned to risk, endure, sacrifice, and work *today,* so they can enjoy greater rewards tomorrow. Ask any successful dieter. Without pain there is no gain (or in the dieter's case, loss).

It would be wonderful if women could learn to see risk as men do—a challenge, an opportunity, a win-some-lose-some proposition—and not be afraid to "go for it." Until we do, indecision and procrastination will continue to hamper us personally and professionally.

Chapter 9

Productivity

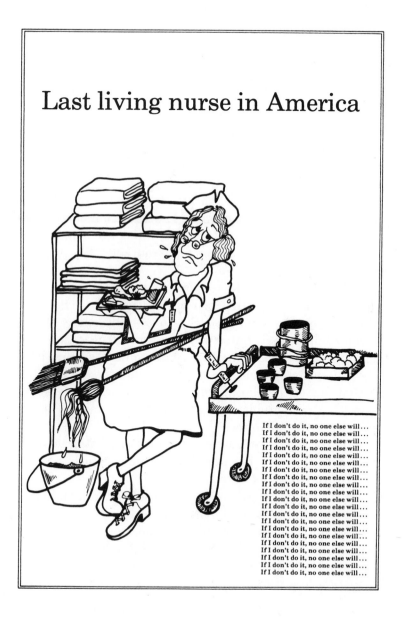

Lᴇᴛ's face it. Nursing needed to be restructured and redesigned. It was about time hospitals began to question whether nurses should be doing *every* task. But suddenly, hospitals began to question whether nurses were actually needed for *any* task.

Today even the word *nurse* seems to be under assault. There are those who use the word so frequently, flippantly, and inappropriately that it has almost lost all meaning. There are others who seem bent on systematically eliminating it from our vocabulary. Let me explain.

As my German shepherd's veterinarian left the examining room, she said, "The nurse will collect the specimen and then you can take Pandora home."

I smiled. I knew there was no "nurse." I thought it was kind of cute. There was no deception intended. None taken.

When dealing with human health care, however, it's a different story. Every day patients are deceived. And the deception is deliberate. It happens in clinics, hospitals, extended care facilities, and doctor's offices across the country. People with no formal education and just a smattering of on-the-job training are calling themselves nurses. Their employers don't discourage the practice. They invented it!

We've allowed people to play fast and loose with the title "nurse." It's a practice that concerned the Oregon Board of Nursing so much they sent a letter to all physicians in the state *reminding* them that "nurse" is a protected, legal title.

Sally, a nurse employed by a government agency, has to deal daily with outlying clinics scattered around the state of Texas. The fact that few of the clinics employ any nurses at all is a constant source of concern and irritation to her. As she says, "The clinics are staffed by 'artificial' nurses."

Recently, she called one of the clinics and asked to speak to the doctor in charge. The receptionist said he was busy but she would put her through to his nurse.

"Don't give me that," Sally curtly replied. "You and I both know there is no nurse employed by your clinic!"

There was a moment of silence. The receptionist hemmed and hawed. Finally, she connected Sally with the doctor.

Another nurse reported that her extended care facility had just instituted a policy requiring nurse's aides to wear *whites and caps.* If you think that was done to reassure confused patients, I have a bridge I'd like to sell you.

I was talking with Ruth Bashford, Executive Director of the Delaware Nurses Association, about this problem.

"Well, let me tell you what happened to me!" she exclaimed.

Because of changes in her organization's health care insurance, she had gone to a new physician for her annual physical exam. She was perched on the examining table waiting for the doctor when a woman waltzed into the room and said, "My name is Such-and-Such. I'm Dr. So-and-So's nurse."

Well, you know how chummy we nurses are. Right away Ruth said, "Oh, I'm a nurse too!" Trying to strike up a conversation she asked, "Where did you go to school?"

The woman looked at her and said, "No, you don't understand. I'm *Doctor So-and-So's* nurse. I didn't go to nursing school."

"Ruth, what did you do?" I asked.

"I changed doctors!" she replied.

Then I asked her if she could confirm a rumor. I had been told that nurses in a hospital in Michigan had been issued new name tags with the "RN" removed. The professional staff had been diluted to such an extent that administration was afraid patients would be alarmed when they began to realize how few and far between "real nurses" were in their facility. So they stripped the nurses of any identifying marks.

The nurses were outraged. Administration refused to budge.

So guess what the nurses did. They pinned on their caps!

Ruth hadn't heard the story but she was a good friend of the executive director of the Michigan Nurses Association. She said, "I'll call her and get back to you." A little while later the phone rang, "It's true!"

Then she told me the rest of the story. The nurses sought legal counsel. It turned out Michigan law requires professional staff be identified so new name tags had to be issued. The law, however, varies from state to state.

Another nurse I talked with told me her hospital had removed the word *nurse* from job titles and was experimenting with the title "Health Care Provider." There were different levels from I to IV. Do you think a physician would surrender his title of "doctor" to become a "health care provider" at any level? Not on your life! Nurses shouldn't surrender either.

I remember when one of nursing's notables suggested changing "nurse" to "Clinical Decision Maker." That's a mouthful. Thank goodness we didn't swallow it.

I know, a rose by any other name may smell as sweet, but a nurse by any other name stinks.

"The longer the title, the less important the person."

That's Tip 266 of 500 secrets for success from John M. Capozzi, author of *Why Climb the Corporate Ladder When You Can Take the Elevator* (Penguin Books, 1994).

That's why I like *nurse.*

Words are powerful. Language is all we have. It can be used to clarify or confuse, to define or deceive. That's why we must work together to make sure "nurse" doesn't continue to dissolve into something meaningless or become archaic.

For a moment let's forget all the flap about whether nursing is or is not a profession. Let's just roll up our sleeves and get down to business.

The formula for any successful business is to find a need and fill it—at a healthy profit, of course. Finding needs to fill isn't difficult. Need is everywhere. And nurses pride themselves on being "need-meeters."

Much like weed-eaters, which whirl around with lightning speed mowing down weeds, nurses like to mow down needs. "Show me a need, *any* need, and I'll meet it!"

As indiscriminate need-meeters, we whirl around taking care of everything for everybody everywhere. Remember the nurse who quipped, "Nursing is what nurses do. And nurses do everything!" His words sum up nursing's greatest productivity problem.

No one can do everything. Not even a nurse. Nurses have to recognize that although we are capable of doing almost *anything,* we simply cannot do *everything.*

As long as nursing remains vague about its own mission and goals, it can be easily distracted and exploited. For years our reluctance to put a respectable dollar value on our time made us a cheap, plentiful, and versatile source of labor subsidizing almost every other department in the hospital.

Much of our time is still devoured facilitating the productivity of others. We've all been called on to cover pharmacy, take up the slack for dietary kitchen, transport patients to x-ray, act as security guards, make minor mechanical repairs, run to central supply, clean rooms, and deliver everything from mail to babies.

Occasionally such diverse chores are really nursing incognito.

We straighten up a patient's room while we unobtrusively observe and interview. We transport seriously ill patients for their safety. We gather up dinner trays to keep better tabs on a particular patient's nutrition.

Most of the time, however, nurses do these chores because "Somebody has to do it" or because "If I don't do it, no one else will." Those are direct quotes from indiscriminate need-meeters in action.

Deciding exactly what services nursing will provide is only half the battle. The other half is deciding what services nursing will *not* provide. Even nice nurses will have to learn to say "no." We have to learn to be "discriminating need-meeters." We have to make conscious choices about *whose* needs we will meet, *which* needs we will meet, *where* we will meet those needs . . . *what* . . . *when* . . . *why* . . . and *how*.

When a large veterans' hospital contacted me to do an "emergency" assertiveness workshop, I laughed. In all my years of teaching assertiveness, I had never heard of an emergency assertiveness workshop.

They were struggling with the nurse shortage. They had stretched their existing staff just about to the breaking point and they wanted me to come in and teach their nurses to just say "no" to nonnursing tasks, which is difficult to do on two counts. First, we are unclear about what is and is not nursing's responsibility, and second, nurses are just terminally helpful, friendly people. We see a problem and we swing into action. We mop it up, fix it up, kiss it, make it better. And while we are distracted by these low-level tasks, be they janitorial or clerical in nature, things that require the critical eye of a professionally skilled nurse are going totally unattended.

While nursing seems to get its kicks messing about in every other department's business, no other department in the hospital is looking out for nursing's business. It is just going undone.

One approach was to have the nurse hierarchy at the VA discuss the problem with other department heads. When made aware of the nurse shortage, those department managers began to make some significant changes. However, the basic problem remained— getting nurses to just say "no."

When asked for examples of nonnursing tasks, nurses tell of defrosting refrigerators, cleaning utility rooms, running errands, chasing supplies, and doing endless paperwork. Every day almost half of the nurse's time evaporates this way.

In one hospital I was told housekeeping would not clean the "dirty dirt." Hospitals deal in dirty dirt. Therefore, the housekeeping department must deal in dirty dirt. Nothing else makes sense.

A pediatric head nurse said peas had been served to the children at lunch. Now peas were rolling all over the floor. She called housekeeping. A janitor came up, leaned on his broom, and announced, "I don't do peas."

I asked the head nurse what she did. She said she didn't know what to do so she began picking up the peas. The mothers of her patients helped.

What's wrong with this picture?

A *professional* nurse whose decisions influence life and death can be buffaloed by a broom jockey with an attitude! The patients' mothers—*customers* who are paying through the nose—are crawling around on their hands and knees picking up peas!

In a large metropolitan hospital, respiratory therapy was ordered twice a day. However, respiratory therapists were only doing one treatment a day. Nurses were doing the second treatment. Then nursing discovered that respiratory therapy was billing the clients for two treatments a day. Nursing sent a bill charging RT for all the nurse hours involved. When RT protested, nursing said simply, "If we do the work, we will collect the revenue." In 24 hours the RT department expanded its coverage. They wanted the revenue, but why should they do the work when the nurses were doing it for free without even thinking it through?

Nurses are busy people, but being busy isn't the same as being productive. Busy or productive? It all depends on how we define:

The Business of Nursing

Productive people know how to mind their own business. Unfortunately, very few nurses have a clear idea of what their business is.

If I asked you to define the business of nursing in 25 words or less, what would *you* say? Go ahead, take a stab at it. I'll wait.

"As nurses our business is _assess patients subjectively and objectively using the nursing process considering psy/soc, culture, age and gender specifications, provide health maintainer._"

Chances are you skipped the above exercise, dismissing the answer as either obvious or impossible. It is neither.

You may have searched your mind for cobwebbed remnants of all those bio-psycho-social-cultural-spiritual-needing-wanting-life span definitions you memorized long ago. You may have come up with a definition similar to one of the following. Let me share some responses from other nurses who have tried to define the business of nursing.

What Is the Business of Nursing?

"Taking care of the sick"

"Alleviating the distress of patients by applying all our knowledge and expertise"

"To provide care for those who are ill and to prevent illness in those who are well"

"The giving of oneself for the care and benefit of others"

"Teaching patients to take care of themselves!"

"Seeing that the needs of a person are taken care of, either personally or through coordination with others—this includes all needs from physical to emotional to spiritual, including family, friends, etc."

"The business of nursing is to do those things that are no one else's business."

"Dealing in health care, not only for the patient but for the family, from admission to discharge—either by physician or death"

"Caring"

"Taking care of patients' and physicians' problems, all of which require a lot of care"

"Providing a mutually agreeable service that assists clients to become functionally independent"

"Taking care of patients in all aspects using knowledge of good health care for both sick and well—it is a profession requiring lots of stamina, love, and knowledge."

"?????"

"Caring for human beings or educating them to care for themselves in an intelligent, efficient, and cost-effective manner"

"Charity—love and faith"

And my personal favorite from Ron Bayless, RN, poet laureate:

"Doing the necessary for the needy, being speedy, and not greedy"

You are bound to find some of the definitions appealing and some appalling. Each has its own merits. Each reflects choices made by the author. Collectively they serve to remind us that there is *no one right answer*.

Choice is the key. Of all the bio-psycho-social-*ad infinitum* needs waiting to be met, nursing has yet to make a conscious, deliberate, and courageous choice.

Examining nursing as a business and not as a duty, calling, or profession may be novel enough to bring new insights to some old problems that have plagued us for years. Although I don't have all the answers, I think I have identified the most important question to ask of nursing today: "What is our business?"

Where do we begin to find an answer to that question? The root of any business definition is the customer. The customer is the *only* reason for any business to exist. It is the customer's wants, wishes, needs, and values that guide the business.

Who is nursing's customer? *The Patient.*

That answer is not wrong, but it is not right either. The patient is just *one* of nursing's customers. Actually very few patients engage nurses directly in a buyer-seller-of-service transaction. Most nurses wholesale themselves to an employer—hospital, doctor, clinic, school, agency. The employer then sells a complex package of products and services to the customer, which includes nursing care.

Who is another of nursing's customers? *The Employer.*

Once nursing wholesales itself to an employer, it loses much control over its practice and utilization. In a sense, the employer "owns" nursing. Bought and paid for, nursing must then bend to the employer's decisions on utilization, practice, deployment, direction, and appropriation.

Nurses are not the only professionals who wholesale themselves. Any doctor or lawyer who gives up private practice for a salaried position must regard the employer as a most important customer.

Nurses who have been taught to focus almost exclusively on the patient and encouraged to strive for professional autonomy are bound to be confused and frustrated by the realities of employment. Our educational background leaves us woefully ignorant of politics, economics, management, and organizational behavior.

Speaking of our educational background, perhaps many of the disputes between nursing education and nursing service would disappear if education looked upon service as its prime customer. For years nursing service has objected to new graduates who are all thumbs and theory. Nursing education simply is not listening to its customer.

The only way to increase our productivity is to know what we are to produce. The only way to know what to produce is to scrutinize our customers—all our customers. We have to know who they are, where they are, and what they want or need or value enough to actually purchase.

An initial description of nursing's customers might be condensed to read:

Who are our customers?	*Everyone*
Where are our customers?	*Everywhere*
What do they value?	*Everything*

When pressed for more details, nurses have produced lists like these:

WHO ARE OUR CUSTOMERS?	WHERE ARE OUR CUSTOMERS?
Patients	In hospitals
Doctors	In waiting rooms
Hospitals	In clinics
Schools	At the health department
Communities	In factories
Government	In schools
Families	In churches
Ill-well, young-old	On the telephone
Industry	In the streets
Nursing service	At home
All creatures great and small	From nurseries to nursing homes

WHAT DO OUR CUSTOMERS VALUE?

Comfort!	Being normal	Efficiency
Independence	Their life	Effectiveness
Mobility	Speedy recovery	Anticipation of needs
Health	Knowledge	Individualized attention
Money	Respect	Expert opinion
Themselves	Privacy	Compassion
Traditions	Nurturance	Dignity
Quality care	Politeness	Not enough!
	Promptness	

Keeping these lists in mind, let's zero in on a few of those what-is-the-business-of-nursing definitions and see what implications they might have if chosen by nursing as its business definition.

The business of nursing is "taking care of the sick."

A wellness buff would have a minor stroke after reading the above definition. But before judging the author too harshly, consider one thing: her definition makes nursing manageable. She does not see nursing as a do-everything-for-everybody-everywhere profession.

She wants to "do one thing and do it right!" That formula has worked well for physicians. They do a good job of meeting a very few specific needs. Some worry that indeed their services are too few and too specific.

Doctors know their business. They fill *a* need. They do not feel compelled to meet *all* needs. They specialize and make a healthy profit by knowing more and more about less and less.

The business of nursing is "to provide care for those who are ill and to prevent illness in those who are well."

This two-pronged approach is more ambitious and less manage-able than just "taking care of the sick." It forces us to divide nurs-ing resources (time, energy, education, personnel), allocating some to care for the sick and others to keep people well.

Most nurses spend their professional lives taking care of the sick. The need is obvious. The money is there. It's tradition!

But traditions are being broken by health maintenance organi-zations that profit when people are well, not when they are sick. Many industrial giants are launching programs to cut their health bills by encouraging healthier lifestyles for their employees, retirees, and dependents. They are sponsoring health fairs, screen-ing for high blood pressure and glaucoma, and using computers to find the best prices among hospitals and physicians.

The business of nursing is "giving oneself for the care and benefit of others."

"Giving oneself" speaks of sacrifice, not success. Once again we see a nurse's confusion between career and charity. We see the diffi-culty many have when it comes to even discussing nursing as a business.

CAUTION, NURSES: Nothing given away is ever appreciated. If you do not place a high value on your time, talent, education, experience, and ability, no one else will either.

Like it or not, in our society the pervading feeling is that as the price increases, so does the value of the service or product.

Designer jeans—same denim, same thread, same fit, same wear. Add a designer's name and double the price.

Health care—same goal, same approach, same information, same treatment. Add a doctor's name and double the price.

People seeking "professional" care expect to pay for it. If they do not have to pay for it, they regard it as unprofessional.

The business of nursing is "seeing that the needs of a person are taken care of, either personally or through coordination with others. This includes all needs from physical to emotional to spiritual, including family, friends, etc."

Beware the "et cetera."

One of the most scathing reviews of an actor was that "he suffered from delusions of adequacy." Every time I hear nurses exhorted to meet *all* needs physical, emotional, and spiritual, I wonder if nurses aren't suffering from "delusions of adequacy."

By refusing to put boundaries on the scope of nursing, we set ourselves up for much frustration and ultimate failure. One nurse and one profession cannot be all things to all people.

The business of nursing is "to do those things that are no one else's business."

I love this definition. When we are asked what nurses do, it enables us to say, "None of your business!"

Actually, it is very descriptive. For years nurses have followed doctors through the health care field, like gleaners, picking up the leftovers. (You may recall that in biblical times gleaning was an acceptable way to survive. After the landowners had harvested a field, gleaners went through gathering up grain left behind.)

Nurses often behave as if doctors owned the health care field and were generous to let nurses pick up anything they didn't want. Come to think of it, doctors often behave that way too.

Today a multitude of health care specialists have joined doctors tramping through the field. Unlike nurses, each group seems to know exactly what it wants to reap.

Nurses continue to trail behind, trying to sustain the profession on leftovers. Many feel our meager existence is threatened.

Gleaners may survive, but they never thrive. Many nurses, tired of gleaning, leave the health care field altogether. Others decide to get up a little earlier in the morning and beat some of those Johnny-come-latelies into the field. Some have actually bought their own fields.

If you find you're in the wrong field, even for the right reasons, you may not survive. If your field is full of weeds, overworked, eroded, or nonproductive, perhaps it is time to change fields. Heaven knows the whole field of wellness seems up for grabs.

The business of nursing is "?????"

For many of us nursing has been reduced to a series of question marks. Is nursing a profession? A job? A career? An art? A science? A dependent, independent, or interdependent activity?

Much like a centipede pondering which foot to put down first, nursing sits immobilized by indecision. Our theorists, philosophers, and leaders need to stop pondering and put a foot down—any foot. It's always better to be limping than paralyzed.

Perhaps you and I can put things in motion by making some decisions of our own. Even though we might not presume to speak for "the profession" or for "the hospital," we might be able to speak for our individual units or departments.

Consider one business definition of nursing that we haven't yet explored. It is simply "caring." Perhaps this single word best encompasses nursing.

If you look up *care* and *caring* in the dictionary, you will find this descriptive phrase: "a disquieted state of blended uncertainty, apprehension, and responsibility." (If that's not synonymous with nursing, what is?)

Another phrase used in the definition of *caring* is "painstaking or watchful attention." Watchful attention—that's why people submit to hospitalization. They need watchful attention.

Painstaking or watchful attention is the very core of nursing. When attention ceases, caring ceases. Nursing ceases. It doesn't matter whether inattention is a result of fatigue, absence, indifference, or ignorance. The result is the same.

If you were to ask your co-workers, "What is our business here on 5-West?", they might think you daffy because the answer is so obvious. "Why caring for patients, of course!" they would reply. "Caring is our business."

Caring is a one-word business definition that says everything or nothing depending on how it is applied. Taking caring from the abstract and putting it into action is a highly complex task.

Even if you cannot speak for the profession, the hospital, or the unit, you can speak for yourself.

"As a nurse, my business is _____

_____

_____."

One nurse wrote the business of nursing is "teaching patients to take care of themselves!" Although she may not be able to convince her profession, employer, or even co-workers to adopt this definition, she can choose to adopt it.

Once her mission becomes teaching patients to care for themselves, her goals are much clearer. Patient teaching is her top priority. She can no longer relegate it to those few chance moments between her "real" nursing chores.

Working for an employer who does not share her values will be counterproductive at best. This nurse will be most satisfied and satisfactory working in areas that promote preventive medicine or focus on patient self-care. She might find a patient educator position most appealing.

If she decides to pursue a degree, her course work will have to reflect her values and priorities if it is to be at all meaningful or productive.

To be most productive she may actually have to leave the hospital. She might be better utilized in public health or as an industrial consultant. If she has an entrepreneurial spirit, she might go into business for herself helping people to stop smoking, control their weight, or manage stress. For a person with this business definition, these are all legitimate extensions of nursing.

At a national conference I sat in on a session titled "The Entrepreneurial Nurse." Nurses were sharing how they had gotten into business. One nurse had become an architectural consultant. It was not a planned career move, it had just evolved.

It all began when she volunteered to serve on her hospital's building committee. Her family was in the construction business.

She had grown up knowing something about building methods and materials.

For 3 years she served on the committee. The result was a nurse-friendly hospital. She thoroughly enjoyed the project and suddenly realized she could fill an important niche—liason between architects and the nurses who had to work in their creations. She became a very successful consultant.

Ironically, she was about to lose her nursing license. The southwestern state where she lived had a practice component. They argued she was no longer a *real* nurse. She didn't feed people, bathe people, medicate people.

Once again nursing was about to cut off its nose to spite its face. This nurse had accomplished more for our profession in her nontraditional role than she ever could have at the bedside. We need to promote diversity, not punish it.

Unlike Paul Harvey, I cannot tell you the rest of the story. I do not know what the outcome was. I only hope she is still an RN and nursing did not banish her.

Until we nurses decide collectively, locally, and individually just what our business is, we cannot increase our productivity.

The choice is ours: caring for the sick . . . keeping people well . . . doing what we are told . . . teaching patients self-care . . . facilitating the work of other professionals. . . .

The decisions we make will shape our educational policies, set our professional standards, guide our daily work, and ultimately determine our future.

Listen to one last nurse's response to "What is the business of nursing?":

> I would like to answer this question with my *only* answer: "Nursing *is* my business. For the past 27 years it has provided me with an excellent income and been most rewarding in every phase."

Nursing is *my* business too. Let's mind our own business.

Chapter 10

Professional Rights and Responsibilities

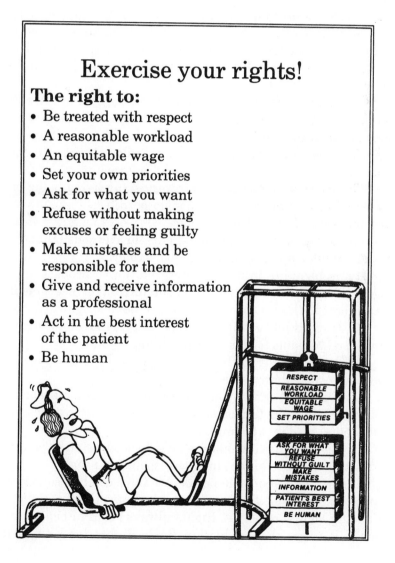

Exercise your rights!

The right to:

- Be treated with respect
- A reasonable workload
- An equitable wage
- Set your own priorities
- Ask for what you want
- Refuse without making excuses or feeling guilty
- Make mistakes and be responsible for them
- Give and receive information as a professional
- Act in the best interest of the patient
- Be human

RESPECT
REASONABLE WORKLOAD
EQUITABLE WAGE
SET PRIORITIES

ASK FOR WHAT YOU WANT
REFUSE WITHOUT GUILT
MAKE MISTAKES
INFORMATION
PATIENT'S BEST INTEREST
BE HUMAN

Rounding a curve on the coastal highway, I spot a rain-drenched hitchhiker. He raises his thumb and smiles hopefully at me.

Chances are he's a poet, a free spirit, or a wandering student who's out to experience life. But there is also a chance that he's a psychotic, a thief, or a murderer. At 50 miles per hour I can't distinguish poets from psychotics, so I don't take chances.

I zip past him and my spirits are briefly dampened by feelings of guilt. *Guilt* . . . because I was reared and educated to be a helper . . . because I was taught to share . . . because I believe in being a Good Samaritan . . . because I'm a "have" and he's a "have not."

I am drawn to a need like a moth to a flame. Unlike the moth, however, I know I can get burned. I *know* better than to pick up hitchhikers. Yet, in that split second our eyes meet, I *feel* compelled to help him. I have to consciously resist the urge to stop.

Why do I feel responsible for every stray living being on life's highway? Because I am a responsible person. It's as automatic as the knee-jerk reflex. When I perceive a person has a need or a right, I feel a responsibility. Your right—my responsibility.

No wonder people take advantage of me!

My problem lies in my misinterpretation of people's needs and rights. They are not synonymous. The hitchhiker needs a ride. He has a right to thumb a ride. He does not have a right to a ride.

My responsibility stops at respecting his right to hitchhike. I am not responsible for his transportation.

You have a right to freedom of speech. I respect your right. I have no responsibility to listen to you.

In a very real sense, your rights are also your responsibilities. You have the right to free speech, but it is *your* responsibility to attract and hold an audience.

I *could* give the hitchhiker a ride. I *could* listen to you. Should I? That's the question that haunts responsible people.

Nurses are responsible people. We have dwelled so long and so hard on our responsibilities, we are often surprised at the prospect of having rights ourselves. Rights always seem to belong to other people. Perhaps that's why Ten Basic Rights for Women in the

Health Professions is the most frequently requested reprint from *STAT.**

To refresh your memory, here are those basic rights:

1. You have the right to be treated with respect.
2. You have the right to a reasonable work load.
3. You have the right to an equitable wage.
4. You have the right to determine your own priorities.
5. You have the right to ask for what you want.
6. You have the right to refuse without making excuses or feeling guilty.
7. You have the right to make mistakes and be responsible for them.
8. You have the right to give and receive information as a professional.
9. You have the right to act in the best interest of the patient.
10. You have the right to be human.

These rights are yours, but acquiring and holding them is *your* responsibility. Not the doctor's. Not the head nurse's. Not the administrator's. Yours.

Let's revisit each of these ten rights and see some of the dilemmas and delights they pose for responsible people.

You Have the Right to Be Treated with Respect

Mutual respect is absolutely essential if there is to be any semblance of a health care *team.* Unfortunately, I am inundated with examples of doctor-nurse interactions in which respect is sorely lacking.

Doctors often behave as if they had a right to humiliate nurses. Nurses often behave as if they had a responsibility to stand there and be humiliated.

> On many occasions while working as an RN/Scrub Assistant we were told that "even a goddamn monkey can be taught to scrub." We were referred to at various times as stupid and slow. My only response was to pout and throw icy stares. (Very effective. Ha ha!)

---

*Chenevert, Melodie: *STAT: Special techniques in assertiveness training for women in the health professions,* ed. 4, St. Louis, 1994, Mosby.

As long as nurses submit to such humiliation, it will continue. Pouts and icy stares are not effective deterrents because they are too easily ignored. You can get the surgeon's attention by clamping a hemostat on his nose or handing him the wrong end of a scalpel, but those actions tend to escalate hostilities, not increase mutual respect.

Any team tortured and humiliated by its "captain" is not a winning team. If you believe teamwork is in the best interest of your patients, you must confront the surgeon.

Give him the phone number of the zoo and walk out. Nurses are not in the monkey business. Either the insulting behavior is discontinued, or the doctor works alone.

It can be done. Here's proof.

One OR supervisor tells of an irascible doctor who had alienated every scrub nurse on her staff with his haughty demeanor, sarcastic speech, and innumerable temper tantrums. At length every veteran scrub nurse absolutely refused to work with him.

A brand-new nurse had just joined the staff, and it was her luckless lot to be assigned to the beast. Within moments he had reduced her to tears. He stormed out of the room and confronted the supervisor. How dare she assign him some bumbling novice!

The supervisor stood toe-to-toe and eye-to-eye with the surgeon and said calmly, "Doctor, there is not a single nurse on my staff who will scrub with you. That new nurse is your last chance. If she won't assist you, no one will." She pivoted and walked away.

Once out of sight, she ducked into the nearest broom closet. Her knees were like jelly, and her heart was beating so fast she thought she would collapse.

The surgeon paused, then reentered the operating room. He proceeded to make the novice into a first-rate colleague. They were a splendid team for years.

Another physician was famous for throwing patients' charts when he became irritated. One day he threw a chart, splattering its contents all over the end of the hall.

The nurse who was accompanying him on rounds immediately knelt to pick it up. From afar the head nurse bellowed, **"Don't pick up that chart!"** The nurse froze. In a quieter tone the head nurse continued, "The doctor dropped the chart, the doctor will pick it up."

The doctor stared at the head nurse in disbelief. Then he stepped over the chart and stomped off the floor.

An hour later he returned and asked for Mrs. So-and-So's chart. The head nurse replied, "It's at the end of the hall where you left it." The doctor retrieved it. He has never thrown another chart—at least not on that floor.

If nurses are to gain respect, we must behave in a "respectable" manner. Respect must be earned. Groveling, cowering, and kow-towing are not actions that command respect.

You Have the Right to a Reasonable Work Load

As a new graduate, I was a head nurse. It was a small unit—10 beds. My "staff" consisted of me and an aide. I was responsible for medications, treatments, charting, rounds with physicians, direct patient care, etc.

I consistently worked overtime and asked to be paid for it. The director of nurses repeatedly stated there was no reason for the overtime, and I shouldn't have to be paid.

Finally, in response to her constant harassment, I only asked to be paid overtime occasionally. Often I went home in tears still feeling I deserved to be paid for what I was doing.

The terms *new graduate* and *head nurse* should be mutually exclusive. They should never be synonymous.

Not only is this new graduate in water over her head, she is going down for the third time. Hearing her cries for help, the director of nurses scolds her for drowning. Instead of throwing a life preserver, she throws stones.

Overtime is not the problem. It is a symptom of the problem. Whether the problem lies within the new nurse or within the hospital system, nothing is being done to correct it.

The young nurse will not be with that hospital long. With this sort of initiation into nursing, she won't be in the profession long. As for the director of nursing, well . . . she obviously lacks organizational management skills every bit as much as the new graduate.

A clinical nurse specialist was hired to spend 30% of her time with the perinatal team. At weekly "team" meetings she was constantly harassed by the physicians who demanded she explain why she was not doing everything a full-time person could do.

She tried reasoning with them. She explained that 30% of a

40-hour week is only 12 hours. One person can only do so much in that short amount of time. But the doctors continued to push and complain.

The meetings exhausted her. Afterward, feeling humiliated and defeated, she retreated to her office to lick her wounds. She began to dread those meetings so much she was thinking of resigning.

Then, at an assertiveness workshop, she learned a new technique called fogging. That's a comical name for a very effective technique. During verbal attacks you stand calmly sifting through the barrage for a small statement that has a bit of truth to it. When the attack subsides, you agree with the tiny truth, and then make your counterproposal.

At the next meeting she sat calmly through the doctors' criticism. Then she looked at them and said, "Gentlemen, you are absolutely right. You do need a clinical nurse specialist full-time. I am prepared to leave the hospital staff and come to work for you directly. For $40,000 a year you can have my undivided attention."

The doctors were speechless. It never occurred to them that if they wanted more service, they would have to pay for it.

In subsequent meetings, if a criticism arose, the nurse just reiterated her offer and smiled.

> I am a nurse administrator in a medical/surgical/psychiatric setting. I am required to function both as a team leader and nursing supervisor.
>
> Recently our part-time psychiatrist who was responsible for the 90-day reviews of patient progress and revision of psychiatric treatment plans resigned. The administration informed me that I would assume this responsibility.
>
> I objected, especially since this would not include a salary raise. I must not have been assertive enough because I was coerced into doing this.

This nurse is one of the multitude of nurses employed by institutions that are generous with responsibilities and stingy with rewards and recognition. Hospitals don't expect nurses to negotiate. They expect them to do as they are told.

And we do!

A skilled, self-respecting professional would negotiate a fee for service or a contract comparable to the one enjoyed by the part-time psychiatrist. Actually, a nurse could probably provide quality service at half the cost and save the hospital a bundle while making herself a fortune. That should make everyone happy. Unfortunately, this nurse works at Ebenezer Scrooge Memorial. They don't want to pay less. They want to pay nothing.

Perhaps this nurse can function adequately as a pseudopsychiatrist. Does the Board of Nursing think so? What about the JCAHO? These factors enter into any negotiation.

If salary cannot be negotiated, work load must be. Before picking up this new responsibility, negotiate exactly what will be put down. Few nurses have the time necessary to absorb such a large and important task. Being team leader and supervisor is bound to keep this nurse busy. If she is to be their "psychiatrist," which do they want to relieve her of: team leading or supervising?

Her last comment about being "coerced into doing this" could be echoed by every overworked nurse. How did they coerce her? Did they chain her to a desk and withhold food and water until she completed those 90-day reviews? Did they beat her? Did they hold her family hostage?

No. They sang a few choruses of the "If-You-Don't-Do-It-No-One-Else-Will Blues." They implied the patients would suffer if she did not do as she was told. They called her sense of duty, loyalty, and professionalism into question. They threatened her with the loss of her "nice-nurse" reputation.

She was not coerced. She was flimflammed.

You Have the Right to an Equitable Wage

After speaking at a national conference, I was taken aside by a woman who objected to my use of the term *wage*. As a nursing instructor she taught her students that "workers earn wages, professionals earn salaries."

Considering the fact that many nurses are required to punch time clocks and are often paid less than unskilled male laborers, I think I'll stick with the word *wage*.

> I have been employed at "St. Ignats" for 9 years. My job title is nursing practitioner. My job responsibilities presently include direct clinical service, staff and student nurse supervision, and program planning. In the past I have had administrative responsibilities and directed staff in-service. I have wanted to upgrade my position for a long time.

About 5 years ago I half-heartedly talked with the director of staffing and recruitment for nursing, stating that I had many more responsibilities than the average staff nurse. I allowed myself to be put off by her reasoning that as the only nurse in my department I would be unable to get a higher position regardless of my responsibilities. I have not spoken with her again about this matter. I would like to try again and this time succeed.

Isn't it amazing how easily nurses are controlled by any statement masquerading as logic. I can hear the director cooing, "Yes, I know you have many more responsibilities than the average staff nurse. But you are the only nurse in your department. You are already at the top. There is no way you can be given a higher position."

Why wouldn't the director's reasoning apply to the head of General Motors or the administrator of the hospital? Because it is not logical. Their salaries reflect the responsibilities they assume. As responsibilities increase, so do reward and recognition—except in nursing.

This director is a master of managerial politics. I know because I was once asked to speak at a conference by that title, and whenever I am asked to speak, I consult a dictionary to look up all the words in the conference theme or title. (I hope people conducting conferences do the same.)

Preparing for that particular conference, I looked up *managerial politics* in my dictionary and explored all ramifications of those two words. I assembled many possible meanings for the phrase. My favorite was "to make and keep submissive by artful and often dishonest practices." Although I am sure the conference organizers did not have that particular combination in mind, that definition captures the director's behavior.

For years this rather exploited nurse has shouldered her share of responsibilities. Now she wants more. She wants the rewards and recognition that should accompany her position. Unlike the head of General Motors and the hospital administrator, however, she is not sure she "deserves" them.

Her lack of confidence in her own worth defeated her 5 years ago when she "half-heartedly" approached the director. Lack of confidence will defeat her again. Salaries, like respect, have to be earned. You have to command them.

After 15 years as a part-time float nurse in a 250-bed hospital, I was offered the position of relief supervisor from 4 P.M. to midnight. I was given a 50-cent-an-hour raise and promised I would be reviewed in 6 months.

Six months passed—no review.

Twelve months passed—no review.

Eighteen months passed—no review.

The director of nursing had multiple personal problems during this time, so I kept making excuses for her delay. But after 18 months, I made an appointment to see her about it.

She said my review had completely skipped her mind. Then, because I was already making "top staff-nurse wages," she wasn't sure a raise was in order. She promised to think about it.

Two weeks later she called me in and offered me a 6-cent raise. Yes! Six cents!!! After performing as a supervisor for a year and a half, she offered me a 6-cent raise.

I resigned my supervisory position at that meeting and returned to being a float nurse. It was one of the most difficult things I have ever done.

Six months later she called me in and offered me $3 an hour over top staff-nurse wages if I would become supervisor again. I happily agreed. I love being a supervisor.

I consider the 6 months I went back to floating the most valuable 6 months of my career. I have to say those were also the hardest 6 months of my life.

Was it worth it? You bet it was!

You Have the Right to Determine Your Own Priorities

If you don't exercise your right to set your own priorities, you will get plenty of exercise attending to other people's priorities.

I wish I had been more assertive when I took my present job— combined clinical and classroom teaching:

Too much work

Too little pay

Too little time to prepare lectures, grade papers, counsel students, meetings, etc.

I like my job, but it's too much to handle, especially when we are expected to get a master's on our own time. I have a husband and young son at home. I feel exhausted much of the work year.

This nurse is caught in the cross-fire of competing priorities. She can't keep everyone happy. Her best bet is to set and honor her own priorities, or she will be pulled apart by other people's unrealistic demands. She needs to accept the fact that other people's priorities are not necessarily her priorities.

Her plight reminds me of a newlywed nurse who used to rise quietly so she wouldn't wake her sleeping husband and tiptoe around the house getting ready for work. When she left at 6:15 A.M. he was still sleeping peacefully. He didn't have to leave for work for a full 2 hours.

Arriving home in the late afternoon, she dashed madly about cleaning and cooking. When her husband arrived home, he dropped into his favorite chair, read the paper, and relaxed. After dinner their evenings were free for romance. Ah, youth!

The young husband never once washed the dishes or performed any other household chore. It never occurred to either of them that he should.

More than a year passed. The nurse found she was too tired for romantic evenings. She fell asleep soon after dinner. In the early morning hours, she began to resent her sleeping husband as she hurriedly dressed for work.

Then one day her husband called it to her attention that a colleague's wife got up at 5:00 A.M. so she could wax the floors before leaving for work. He added, "Maybe you ought to try that."

Something snapped. From that moment on the days of the marriage were numbered.

When the nurse married again, her priorities had changed substantially. She chose a husband who would share the work as well as the fun. They've been happily married almost 20 years.

Passions cool. Priorities change. Important things on one day may be insignificant the next. Just remember, there are no wrong priorities as long as they're *your* priorities.

You Have the Right to Ask for What You Want

This is one right I have considered rephrasing. Nurses are so hesitant to ask for what they *need,* they cannot accept the idea of asking for what they want. It seems too self-indulgent.

For example, a recently widowed nurse with young children found her full-time job and single-parent responsibilities overwhelming. She wanted to reduce her work week to 4 days. Although she could manage on the reduced salary, having a handicapped child made a concurrent reduction in health care coverage unbearable.

For weeks she agonized over her dilemma. Finally she screwed up her courage and made an appointment with the administrator. Preparing for that appointment, she gathered facts, figures, and testimonials. She rehearsed responses to any questions or arguments he might have.

Once in his office she began, "I can only work 4 days a week, but I simply must have full health coverage."

Before she could continue, he said, "Fine."

"What?"

"I said that's fine."

She thanked him and nearly danced out of the office. She kicked herself for not having asked sooner.

Another nurse writes:

> As a part-time relief nurse, I was being sent to every unit in the hospital. The chief of nursing, being an ex-army nurse, felt that *any* nurse should be able to work *any* place needed in the hospital.
>
> One evening she ordered me to go to the emergency room. I went to her office and refused, saying I wasn't knowledgeable or experienced enough to work in that area. She agreed and sent me elsewhere. What a relief!

Happy endings—they are never guaranteed, but you will rarely get what you want unless you ask for it.

✠
_____

You Have the Right to Refuse Without Making Excuses or Feeling Guilty

Whenever a nurse refuses a request or a command from a superior, she feels guilty. She feels guilty even if she is within her rights, even if it is her responsibility to refuse.

Here are two examples in which nurses refused. Backed by knowledge, experience, and hospital policy, they held their ground. They were not comfortable, but they refused to be intimidated.

> As weekend charge nurse, I was ordered to give uncrossmatched blood, but no physician would sign to take responsibility in case of a reaction. I was told to sign—"everything will be okay"—yet not one of the three doctors involved would sign themselves.

Firmly I told the doctors, "No signature. No blood." Later I received an apology and a thanks.

The following nurse is caught in a crunch between a hospital policy and a physician who thinks he is above such policies.

Several weeks ago I received a lab result of a fasting blood sugar of 675 on a diabetic patient who was on insulin. I called the patient's MD who told me to call the patient and tell him to change his insulin dosage.

Hospital policy states we cannot take telephone orders. I informed the MD of this. He became very nasty on the phone, stating nurses were stupid and had stupid rules, etc. About a half hour later he came to the clinic and started to write the order for the insulin increase. Suddenly he decided the patient should be admitted and changed the orders. While there he again made insulting remarks about nurses.

The patient was called and advised to come to the hospital. He remained in the hospital three weeks.

I felt despite the MD's insulting and abusive remarks I had asserted my rights as a nurse and an individual.

It is far better to refuse than capitulate and risk a serious error. Failure to refuse can make you a sorry excuse for a nurse.

You Have the Right to Make Mistakes and Be Responsible for Them

Not surprisingly, it is difficult to get workshop participants to share examples of mistakes they have made. Professionals don't make mistakes. I wish that were true.

A young nurse made a terrible error. She went home sobbing. Unfortunately, the next day was her day off. I said "unfortunately" because I really believe it is like falling off a horse. If you don't get right back up on and ride, you may never darken the door of a hospital again.

While she was home the next day, the doorbell rang. There stood a messenger with a big bouquet of flowers. It was from her fellow nurses on the unit. The card attached read, "We hope today is better than yesterday and we look forward to seeing you Thursday."

Talk about a pivotal moment in a young nurse's career!

How do you treat yourself or a colleague when a mistake is made? Nurses are usually very hard on themselves and on each other.

Although being a professional lessens the chance of error, it does not eliminate the possibility of mistakes. Acknowledging our mistakes is painful but necessary for professional growth.

> When I was working a night shift, I had an LPN, another RN, and an older aide working with me. One night a patient fell and was unconscious on the floor.
>
> I told everybody not to move the patient and started to take vital signs. The older aide said, "We have to move him to bed because we can't have a code on the floor." She started moving him with the LPN's help.
>
> When the doctor came in and saw the patient, he said we should not have moved him because of the possibility of a cervical fracture. And I felt bad.

The nurse in this situation made a grave error. Her mistake was caused by lack of confidence in her own professional judgment. She allowed an aide to usurp her authority. If the patient is injured, it is the nurse, not the aide, who must accept the responsibility.

The incident is symptomatic of a much larger problem. Not only does this nurse need to review basic first aid, she needs to gain the skill and confidence necessary to effectively exert the authority of her position and her profession. Sometimes I think we need a nationwide confidence-building program for nurses.

✠ ――――――――――――――――――――――――――――――――――――――

You Have the Right to Give and Receive Information as a Professional

Nurses have both the right and the responsibility of keeping doctors informed about their patients. Yet many nurses dread telephoning physicians because they have received so many tongue lashings. Here's how one nurse solved the problem:

> A doctor was yelling over the phone, using abusive language, saying nothing really pertinent to this patient's care.
>
> Amid the yelling I said, "I can see you're upset. I'm going to hang

up the phone and call you back in 5 minutes. I hope we can discuss your patient's problem calmly."

She hung up. Five minutes later she called him back. Their conversation was polite and productive.

> I'm a public health nurse. When visiting an elderly gentleman who was bedridden and cared for totally by his wife, I found he had rales in his lungs, a temperature, and irregular respirations.
>
> I phoned his doctor who said, "Well, what do you expect me to do about it? He's dying!"
>
> I said, "What you do about it is your responsibility. But it is my responsibility to inform you of changes in the patient's condition."
>
> His tone mellowed and he offered to visit the gentleman at home. I was in shock. Assertiveness could be a dangerous thing for me to know!

The public health nurse exercised her right in a very responsible manner.

You Have the Right to Act in the Best Interest of the Patient

Often nurses have to act in the best interest of their patients because the patients cannot speak for themselves.

> I work as a staff nurse in a hospital OB nursery. One of the baby's bilirubin tests was quite high, and I was anxious to report this to the doctor so treatment could be started.
>
> Well, the doctor arrived and did nothing about this situation. I knew this was wrong but could not say to him that such a thing could not be left for another day.
>
> The next morning testing showed the bilirubin level even higher. The physician on call reprimanded the nurse instead of the other physician.

A nurse too intimidated to speak up for a helpless newborn deserves a reprimand. She also deserves a desensitization program to help her overcome her pathological fear of doctors before it becomes fatal . . . for one of her patients.

Then there are times when the nurse must act in the best interest of a patient because a doctor refuses to do so. Although we always hope for the best, it is wise to be prepared for the worst. Here is one of the worst situations I have ever encountered:

> An ambulatory middle-aged man in respiratory distress came into the ER of our private local hospital with his wife. He did not have a local MD, and after the initial history, I placed a call to our front floor to see if any of the attending doctors were in the hospital.
>
> I was told that Dr. *K* was in the house, and they would tell him of the problem, and he would come back and see the patient. I made the patient comfortable and began talking with the family.
>
> Dr. *K* arrived, and his first question to the patient as he stood in the waiting room of the ER was "Do you have insurance?" The patient replied he did. He said he was employed by a local gas station that carried ——— insurance for their employees.
>
> Dr. *K* replied that that insurance wouldn't cover hospitalization and the medical "won't even begin to pay my bill!" With that he turned and left the ER.
>
> The patient and his wife looked at me. Then they left also.

The doctor's behavior is abominable. The nurse's behavior is inexcusable. More accurately, it is her lack of behavior that is inexcusable.

Caught up in this situation, most of us would be left standing with our mouths open. The doctor would be out of sight before we could gather our wits about us. The doctor got away, but the patient shouldn't have.

This dramatic example is excellent for role play. It helps nurses think on their feet and prepares them for some bad situations in advance. In workshops wonderful responses have emerged ranging from one earth-shattering bellow, "Freeze, Buster!" to an "Oh, boy, I've been waiting for something like this ever since I entered law school. Now let me see if I am quoting you correctly, doctor. . . ."

One acting nurse turned to the acting patient and said, "Thank goodness that quack didn't lay a hand on you. Now I'll get you a *real* doctor."

Another pantomimed picking up the telephone and saying, "Hello, Security Department? There's a mad man impersonating Dr. *K*. Yes, he was just here in the emergency room. I think you will be able to catch him. He's wearing. . . ."

All kidding aside, if you were the responsible person, how would you get proper medical attention for this patient?

You Have the Right to Be Human

I was faced with a situation a few months ago where I thought I was being assertive but evidently did not come across that way. I had identified a key employee (male) as being alcoholic after he was referred to me for evaluation by one of our executive vice presidents.

I reported back to the VP that he was alcoholic. The VP in turn spoke to another officer of the company, and then called me for a meeting to make a decision as to any action to be taken.

As we have a loose "Employee Assistance Program" and I am the resource person to contact, I was under the impression I would be handling this case. Instead, I was told they would counsel this man as I was a female (he would have trouble relating) and "just the nurse."

I maintained that I was qualified through many alcoholism courses and counseling courses and Rutgers Summer School. This meeting lasted 2 hours, and as I was confident in my abilities to handle the matter, I attempted to maintain an assertive manner without being intimidated by the presence of the vice presidents.

It was concluded that they would counsel this man. They attempted to do this for a few months without success and finally sent him to me. This man is now one of our key employees again. But if I perhaps had been more assertive, he would have received the proper treatment much sooner.

Here is a nurse who did everything right. She was professional, persistent, and prepared. It's not her fault that she is "female" and "just a nurse." That's part of her humanness.

Because of her success with this employee, I don't think those VPs will ever dismiss her so lightly again. She has earned the respect she needs to get future jobs done. This example is a triumph.

Isn't it sad she is still haunted by thoughts that she should have done more? She shouldn't have to apologize for being human. None of us should.

Chapter 11

Problem Solving

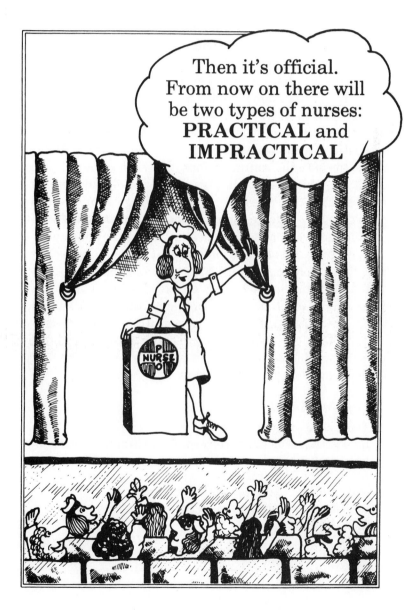

Tʜɪs is a dickens of a time to be in nursing. It is the best of times and the worst of times. On one hand, we seem to be making great strides toward autonomy. On the other hand, we are so confused we don't even know what to call ourselves.

Even if we could gather all 2+ million nurses together and vote on the issues confronting us, we would never get a unanimous vote. If we wait for that impossibility to occur, problems will overrun our profession. It's not bad decisions that will undo nursing, it's the lack of decisions.

When I look back at my over 30-year stint in nursing, I am dismayed to see the same problems cropping up again and again. I find consolation in Edna St. Vincent Millay's words, "Life is not one damn thing after another, it's the same damn thing over and over."

Writing in his classic *The Courage to Create,** Rollo May discusses the painful contradiction of having to be fully committed yet all the while aware that we might possibly be wrong. He goes on to say that "the need for creative courage is in direct proportion to the degree of change the profession is undergoing."

Much of problem solving lies in having the courage to choose a solution from dissenting opinions. The heights we reach will depend more on our courage than anything else.

In effect this entire book is an exercise in problem solving. *Pro-Nurse Handbook* touches on problems ranging from procrastination to productivity, from recruitment to burnout, from exercising rights to facing responsibilities. This chapter is designed to help you solve problems not covered elsewhere in the book. Each section will cover one of the following:

Ten problem-solving tips

Think before taking action.
Be selective. Don't try to solve every problem that comes your way.
Keep goal-oriented.
Activate the 80/20 rule.
Make the best use of the world "as is."
Look for the opportunity hiding behind every problem.
Take the offense.

---

*May, Rollo: *The courage to create,* New York, 1976, W.W. Norton, p. 13.

Learn to negotiate.
Make sure the solution matches the problem.
Expect success.

Think Before Taking Action

There are a half-dozen steps to most problem-solving attempts:

1. Define the problem (preferably in terms of need).
2. Generate a list of possible solutions.
3. Choose one.
4. Implement it.
5. Evaluate the outcome.
6. If the outcome is unsatisfactory, choose another solution or redefine the problem.

Here is a colorful example of the problem-solving process in action. A few years ago a dead whale washed up on the beach. The townspeople walked around the huge carcass trying to figure out how to dispose of it.

First, they tried to drag it back into the sea, but it was so heavy they couldn't budge it. Then someone suggested they cut the carcass into more manageable pieces. That sounded reasonable so they all rushed home to get their chain saws. Unfortunately, the saws just bounced off the whale's tough skin leaving barely a scratch.

By this time the carcass was beginning to decay. The people were becoming more desperate. Someone suggested they stuff the whale with dynamite and blow it apart. *(Moral: Desperate people are not responsible people.)*

Well, they dynamited the critter. It rained whale for miles. Do you have any idea how much damage a flying 20-pound chunk of decaying whale flesh can do?

When the air cleared, the townspeople really had something to blubber about. The bulk of the carcass remained intact on the beach, but now the landscape was splattered with putrifying fragments. *(Moral: Some solutions are worse than the problems.)*

Finally, they decided to send for some sort of derrick to hoist the whale up and drop it out over the ocean. While waiting for the big equipment to arrive, the tide came in and carried the carcass away. *(Moral: Time and tide wait for no derrick.)*

✠
_____

Be Selective. Don't Try to Solve Every Problem That Comes Your Way

Don't be overzealous when it comes to tackling problems. Pause. Make sure the problem is yours or that you are the optimal person to solve it.

Keep a close reign on your good intentions. If the problem actually belongs to someone else, you won't have the authority to enact a lasting solution, and if the problem's owner does not fully endorse your solution, failure is inevitable.

Providing solutions to someone else's problems is often a thankless task. The world is full of ungrateful little twits who will criticize rather than commend your efforts.

As Clare Boothe Luce said, "No good deed goes unpunished."

If at first glance it appears you are the *only* person willing or able to deal with a problem, look again. Something is amiss.

Practice conservation. Concentrate your efforts on the very few problems that really deserve or require attention. Many nurses find their own problems raging out of control because they diverted all their resources into solving other people's problems.

✠
_____

Keep Goal-Oriented

Many nurses find themselves plunging headlong through one helter-skelter day after another. They find that other people's schedules and priorities constantly override their own. They work hard but accomplish little. Their efforts consistently exceed their results.

These nurses are suffering from *goal deficiency,* an acute or chronic disease that has reached epidemic proportions. Symptoms include:

1. Indecision
2. Confusion
3. Frenzied activity
4. Lack of accomplishment
5. Desire to be told what to do and where to go
6. Growing resentment

At the onset of such symptoms, nurses have a tendency to step up their activity. Much like the oft-quoted observer of a bungled military operation said, "Having lost sight of our objective, we redoubled our efforts."

It's not the lack of effort but the lack of goals that keeps successes few and far between.

Basically you need two sets of goals: long haul and short run. Your long-haul goals reflect your life's grand plan. What grand plan? If you don't have one, grab pencil and paper and head for a quiet spot where you can do some uninterrupted thinking.

Write answers to the following questions:

1. What do I want to accomplish in my lifetime?

   _____

2. What do I want to be doing 2 years from now?

   _____

   Five years from now?

   _____

3. If these were my last 6 months on earth, how would I live them?

   _____

"What do I want to accomplish in my lifetime?"

Stumped? Someone has commented that we spend more time planning our vacations than planning our lives. Life just "happens."

A good way to find the answer to this question is to write your own obituary. I know that sounds morbid but it doesn't have to be, because you are free to pick the time, place, and method of your demise. You can die at age 110 driving a Lamborghini in the Indy 500 or at 99 while singing your latest hit on MTV.

Read the obituaries in your local paper. You will see that you can live to be 100 and they can still put your whole life in two paragraphs. That's all you need to write: two paragraphs.

This is the ultimate in being goal-oriented. It will surprise you how many of the decisions that are giving you ulcers or headaches will suddenly be made automatically because they either are or are not in line with your overall lifetime achievement goals.

This exercise can help you decide whether to enroll in college or buy steamship tickets, volunteer to help the Red Cross or learn to tap dance, have a baby or run for political office.

Implicit in this issue is determining what you want to accomplish in your *professional* lifetime. You may need to change jobs or careers if your real obituary is to read properly.

"What do I want to be doing 2 years from now? Five years from now?"

A man wrote to an advice columnist saying he wanted to go to medical school but lamented the fact that he was already 35 years old. He worried that when he began his practice, a full 7 years from now, he would be 42 years old.

The columnist wrote back asking, "And how old will you be in 7 years if you don't go to medical school?"

All of us are getting older. Some of us are getting better. What about you? Are you spending time or investing it?

"If these were my last 6 months on earth, how would I live them?"

If you're leading a cluttered, crowded life and find it difficult to set priorities, try asking yourself the question posed by British critic F. L. Lucas, "Is it worth the amount of life it will cost?"

If you knew you had only 6 months left, I'll wager you would make a lot of changes. You would simply refuse to waste time and energy on people, places, or things that were unimportant.

The connection between daily activities and the sum total of life's accomplishments is easily lost. That's why it is so important to ask yourself these questions at regular intervals. Remember, what you do in the short run determines what you accomplish in the long haul.

In workshops I often ask nurses to write down one of their personal or professional goals. Most stare at their scratch paper, pens immobilized. "Come on," I coax, "just write down one thing that would make your personal or professional life more satisfying." When they still hesitate I ask them to write down something they *wish* were different in their personal or professional lives. That opens the floodgates. Wishes are so much easier to articulate than goals.

"I wish I were thinner!"
"I wish I had my degree."
"I wish I had more weekends off."
"I wish administration would listen to the nurses."
"I wish I were rich."
"I wish I could speak French."
"I wish I could be promoted."
"I wish I could find a husband."

"I wish I could take a trip around the world."
"I wish . . ."

Because it's easier to be a dreamer than a doer, lots of nurses have dreams, but few have goals. What's the difference between a dream and a goal? A *workable* plan.

Many of us are reluctant to admit that making dreams come true has little to do with luck and lots to do with hard work: our own hard work and no one else's. "But let us learn if nothing else that hard work in the absence of goals and workable plans to achieve them remains just that—hard work."*

If you're tired of hard work that doesn't seem to be getting you anywhere, try this next exercise. Take a moment to compile your own wish list. Then select one of your fondest wishes and complete the following:

One thing I want that would make my *personal* or *professional* life more satisfying is _____.

1. What do I need to do to get what I want?

   _____

2. What am I *willing* to do to get what I want?

   _____

3. How will getting what I want affect my life?

   _____

4. Who can I count on to help me get what I want?

   _____

5. What might I do to sabotage myself so I don't get what I want?

   _____

The key to achievement is developing a workable plan specific to each of your goals. For example, say I would like to lose 10 pounds. What do I need to do? Cut calories and start exercising. What am I willing to do? Neither! Therefore, being thinner is a dream, not a goal. I am unwilling to do what is necessary.

---

*Henning, Margaret and Jardim, Anne: *The managerial woman,* New York, 1988, Doubleday.

It's that second question of what I am *willing* to do that separates dreams from goals, fantasies from realities. Nurses wish they were everything from medical missionaries to ballet dancers, but once they ask themselves the questions in this exercise, they quickly see how rare workable plans are. Most are unwilling or unable to do what it takes to make their dreams come true.

For years I've dreamed of owning a house on the Oregon coast. I grew up in Iowa, and when I saw the ocean, I thought I had died and gone to heaven.

Using this exercise I converted that dream into a goal. I developed a workable plan including a special savings account and a subscription to the coastal newspaper. I got a realtor and began learning about the pros and cons of owning vacation property.

The third question is pivotal. "How will getting what I want affect my life?" If you appear to reach a dead end because you are unwilling to do what is necessary, this question may breathe new life into your dream or goal.

For instance, before abandoning my goal of losing 10 pounds, I asked myself how being thinner would affect my life. The benefits held great promise, so I pledged to undertake both diet and exercise.

(In the case of owning ocean property, this question had the opposite effect. The responsibilities, risks, and realities of long-distance ownership would have a negative impact on my life. Turning my dream into a plan may help me to avoid turning my dream into a nightmare.)

"Who can I count on to help me get what I want?" After years of sedentary snacking, I didn't think I could count on myself to lose weight. That's why I enrolled in Weight Watchers and an aerobic exercise class. My husband rallied and joined me in both dieting and exercise.

Surrounding yourself with people who have similar goals increases your chance of success. Avoiding people who don't share your goals will also increase your chance of success. Look at the people who surround you at home and at work. Who can you count on? Who can you convert?

"What might I do to sabotage myself?" I may postpone getting started, succumbing to the "someday syndrome." I may convince myself I am not really fat, I am just short for my weight. I may tell myself I am too busy to exercise. I may neglect my diet because the holidays are approaching or company is coming or any of a hundred other excuses.

This five-question exercise can be used for any of those wish-list items nurses named: getting a college degree, speaking French, improving communications, getting a promotion, finding a husband, becoming rich, or taking a trip around the world.

Occasionally it's possible to achieve two goals with one plan. For nurses who want to be married and rich, Joanna Steichen, a psychotherapist in New York, teaches a course titled, "How to Marry Money." Her qualifications? She is the widow of a wealthy photographer who was 50 years her senior.

Workable plans—what do you need to do? What are you willing to do? How will your life be affected? Who can help you? How might you sabotage yourself?

This simple exercise can also help our profession delineate dreams from goals. For example, nursing wants to be accepted as a "profession." What does nursing need to do? It needs to develop an organized body of specialized knowledge, a code of ethics, standards of practice, consistent educational guidelines, a commitment to research, and peer review.

What is nursing *willing* to do? Therein lies the rub. To date nursing has been either unwilling or unable to meet society's minimal criteria for professions. A blatant shortcoming is in nursing's educational preparation. Professions require professional education that is normally above and beyond the baccalaureate level. So far nursing hasn't even risen to that lowest baseline: the baccalaureate degree.

Nursing educational problems have plagued us long enough. It's time to decide whether acceptance as a profession is worth the effort or not. Either way, making a decision will break us free to pursue goals instead of dreams.

Activate the 80/20 Rule

Long ago and far away, an Italian economist named Pareto spoke of an 80/20 rule. Loosely translated, his rule says that if all items or tasks are listed, 80% of the value, satisfaction, or results will come from 20% of the list.

For example, 80% of the sales come from 20% of the customers, 80% of the sick leave is used by 20% of the employees, 80% of the prescriptions repeat 20% of the drugs, and my own personal favorite, 80% of the dirt is on 20% of the floor.

It's true. Look at your kitchen floor. There is usually a distinct path of dirt. If you grab your mop and take a swipe down that path, in a couple of minutes your kitchen floor will be 80% cleaner. If you drop to your knees and wipe every inch of the floor, you will invest 80% more time but only increase the cleanliness 20%.

By learning 20% of the drugs, procedures, laboratory tests, diets, diseases, and interventions, students can acquire 80% of what they need to know. Of course, if you want to pass, you have to study the *right* 20%.

Generalists master the 20% that is applicable 80% of the time. Specialists master the additional 80%, knowing full well they will only be using it 20% of the time.

If you have 10 tasks to do for a patient, two of them will make 80% of the difference. When schedules are tight or tempers short, it is important to know which two those are.

Admitting we can't meet everyone's every need encourages us to concentrate on high-priority needs. Who determines which needs have highest priority? Each individual. That's why accurate, open communication is imperative.

If the doctor's highest priority is to get the patient's signature on the surgical consent form and he finds it undone, he will be irritated. The fact that all sorts of other good things were done for his patient will not appease him. If the patient desperately wants a shampoo but doesn't get it, he will complain about the lousy care at this hospital in spite of everything else done for him. If the nurse sees predischarge teaching as the most important thing for a particular patient but is unable to get around to it, she will leave work feeling frustrated. Her lack of accomplishment in that one area will obscure her many accomplishments in other areas.

The easiest way to determine priority is to *ask* those involved. One postpartum nurse gives her new parents a dozen index cards, each with a different heading like feeding, bathing, immunizations, and the like. Couples then select topics they wish to have the nurse discuss with them. They leave the hospital raving about the personalized attention they received because *their* needs were met.

Another good example of the 80/20 rule in action is the unit hostess concept. Some units have taken especially sharp volunteers and made them hostess for the day. In other hospitals this is now a salaried position.

The job of the unit hostess is to cruise the halls. Patients know that every 10 to 15 minutes the hostess will pass by their door. If they need fresh water, the TV adjusted, or the blinds opened, the hostess takes care of it. If they need a nurse, the hostess finds their primary care-giver.

What they found happened after they instituted the hostess program was that call lights stopped lighting. Eighty percent of the time patient requests could be handled by a nonprofessional, nontechnical person.

You know what it is like when you are so busy you can't see straight. Call lights are going on up and down the hall. Since you have no way to tell which light signals something important, you just drop everything and make a mad dash.

When you enter the patient's room, he says something like, "I dropped my pencil. I don't see it anywhere. Do you see my pencil?"

And there you are crawling around under the bed retrieving a pencil when you should be at the other end of the hall jump-starting a heart. It is not a good use of a professional nurse's time.

These days when acuity is high, staff is short, and money is tight, we all need to be extremely creative in implementing the 80/20 rule.

Imagine you find yourself working on a hospital unit that is fraught with problems. Morale is low and turnover high. Sometimes the sheer number of problems immobilizes people. Knowing you can't solve all the problems may keep you from solving any.

If you have 10 outstanding problems, which one should you tackle first? *Ask!* Ask your co-workers, "If you could change just one thing on this unit, what would it be?" Listen closely and you'll find one or two problems consistently emerging as high priority. Solving the top two problems may improve morale so much that everyone is able to live with the other eight.

All too often management misreads employees' needs and priorities. They may spend lots of time and money correcting eight problems and only improve the situation 20%. They made a great effort. They just don't understand why they didn't get great results.

Efficiency experts help clients identify and concentrate on that 20% that yields an 80% return. Therefore, their clients can make wise investments whether in terms of time, money, personnel, or effort. Now you know their secret too.

✠
_____

Make the Best Use of the World "As Is"

> If only taxes weren't so high . . .
> If only the paint weren't peeling . . .

If only it didn't rain so much . . .

If only I had a child . . .

If only everyone would stop smoking . . .

If only doctors would respect nurses . . .

If only there were a college in town . . .

We've all played the if-only game. Some of us play it to excess. We spend all our time wishing things were different instead of working with things as they are.

Nurses who base their expectations and actions on a world as it *should be* or *ought to be* rather than on the world as it *is* are destined for frustration and failure.

The world "as is" runs on cash.

The world "as is" is an extremely political place, and yet most nurses have an aversion to anything that smacks of politics.

In the world "as is" I can find no evidence of reason or logic operating anywhere on this planet. I defy you to point out a single example. All you have to do is watch the evening news. Yet our excuse for not taking action is often, "It wouldn't be reasonable" or "It isn't logical."

Learn the system. Use it. It might not seem like much, but it's all we've got.

Look for the Opportunity Hiding Behind Every Problem

Listening to the president of one state's nursing association present their new nurse practice act, I was struck by her constant referral to the nurse as "he." For me, that's like listening to fingernails grating on a blackboard.

Nursing is a woman's profession—*97% female*. To deny that fact not only causes problems, it prevents us from seeing the opportunities.

Instead of cursing the difficulties presented by a predominantly female work force, think of the advantages. Women work harder, longer, and cheaper than men. They are more interested in relationships than reward or recognition. After the age of 45, a Metropolitan Life Insurance Company study showed that *male* employees registered more disability days than female employees. Many corporate studies have demonstrated that older female workers are more dependable, have lower turnover rates, better attendance records, stay on the job longer, and do as much work as their younger counterparts. To top it all off, few women ever collect any pension benefits.

"The *Real* Female Advantage" is the title of an article that appeared in the April 1995 issue of *INC* magazine. A study of 1000 managers revealed that ". . . women don't manage different from men after all—they manage better."

Lawrence A. Pfaff & Associates had evaluations done by people who reported to the managers and the people to whom the managers reported. The results?

> "In every one of the 20 categories showing a statistically significant difference between women and men, both bosses and employees gave female managers higher scores. What's more, the largest performance gaps between women and men were not in 'soft' skills such as communications and teamwork but in areas like planning and decisiveness. Sorry, guys."

Of course, there are some problems associated with a predominantly female staff. One is that women still carry 90% or more of the responsibility for child care in our culture. Attitudes on this subject are changing, but behavior isn't.

Over half the mothers of preschoolers are gainfully employed, and their number grows daily. Two-income families are becoming the rule instead of the exception. When both mother and father are working, a sick child is more than an inconvenience, it can be a crisis. That's why some hospitals not only provide on-site day care for well children but for sick children as well.

Here is how a problem turned into an opportunity and actually provided solutions for more than one problem:

> We have a 20-bed pediatric unit in a 300-bed community hospital. We started to experience a decreased pediatric census in the mid-1980s. Our nurses were being floated to med-surg every day.
>
> We had to think of some way to maintain the integrity of our pediatric unit and to retain the expertise of our nurses. Our first project was a Sick Bay Program that offers day care for sick children of working parents right on our inpatient unit. In 1988 it was approved by the New York State Department of Health. It was so successful we even marketed our Sick Bay Policy and Procedure Manual to raise revenue.
>
> We continued brainstorming ways to fill our pediatric beds. We asked our pediatricians what they would like. They asked for a pedi-

atric outpatient program where children could come to our unit to obtain specimens, rehydration, IV meds, and other less-than-24-hour-stay problems. With the help of administration and our billing department we started an outpatient program on our inpatient unit in 1990.

Our 20-bed unit now has a comprehensive pediatric service of inpatients, outpatients, SDSP, and sick bay clients. Our pediatric nurses no longer have to float. Our turnover rate is minimal.

Whenever I talk to nurses about looking for opportunities hiding behind problems, I can see the skepticism in their eyes. To tired, frustrated, apprehensive, disgruntled nurses it sounds like empty-headed optimism.

Nurses, like most human beings, are quick to spot problems and slow to spot opportunities. So I have them make a list of all the threats and problems they see facing nurses and nursing today.

Burnout	Apathy
Lack of Unity	Disorganization
Low Self-Esteem	Service Occupation
Resistance to Change	Turf Wars
The Economy	DRGs
Politics	Cost Containment
Outmoded Stereotypes	Politicians!
Unrealistic Public Expectations	Misinformation
Entry into Practice	Media
Aging	Lack of Autonomy
Technology	AIDS

Then I ask them to look at the list and see if they can turn any of these problems into an opportunity.

Take politics and politicians. We can learn to play their game. We can run for office. We can become advisors and interpreters so politicians make good decisions. We can campaign and contribute money so nurse-friendly, health-care–smart people are elected.

Disorganization? Lack of unity? We can join one or more of the 70 nursing organizations or associations. And not just pay dues, but actively participate.

Misinformation? Outmoded stereotypes? We can inform the public by teaching and counseling, writing for newspapers and popular magazines, participating in community health fairs, becoming reliable sources of information for journalists, and developing positive relationships with the media.

You get the idea. The next time you're fretting about something, turn it inside out and upside down and shake out the opportunities.

✠

Take the Offense

Be a TOAD. That's an acronym for Take Offensive Action, Dummy!

Nice nurses reading this book will need reassurance that there is quite a difference between being offensive and taking the offense. Think about offense as it's used in sports. Teams alternate playing defense and offense.

In the game of life nurses have spent almost all their time on defense. We have struggled to keep other professionals from gaining ground on us. All the while the opposing players have been chanting, "Push 'em back, Push 'em back, *WAY* back!"

No wonder nurses haven't made many points. To score, we have to grab the ball and run. We have to play offensively.

There are some "offensive" nurses in Oregon—nurse practitioners who acquired prescriptive privileges and went into private practice. At first the physicians weren't very concerned. They expected the nurses to disperse among the rural poor. But some of those nurses had the nerve to open up offices right next door to the doctors in downtown Portland!

Most doctors would be surprised because that's not the sort of future that they have envisioned for nurses. A national cross-section of physicians polled in a 1982 Harris survey said that by 1990 nurse practitioners and physician's assistants would have more responsibility for initial diagnosis and treatment of the rural and urban poor, children and pregnant women, the elderly, and the chronically ill.

Reading between the lines, physicians evidently saw themselves caring for the rural and urban *rich,* adult men, nonpregnant women, the nonelderly, and the acutely ill. No offense, docs, but nurses are getting tired of being expected to take care of your non-profitable patients. If that sounds crass and flagrantly mercenary, it probably is.

Honestly, I am not advocating abandoning the young, old, poor, or chronically ill. I just want to emphasize that nurses need a financially healthy mix of patients every bit as much as those other health professionals do if we are to stay in business.

A nurse who is well compensated by eight of her patients can afford to donate her services to two who cannot pay for care. Unfortunately, nurses expect to eke out a living on two paying clients while donating their services to eight who cannot pay.

A nurse entrepreneur who owns a multimillion dollar agency was recently asked to consult with nursing leaders on a growing problem. It seems there are over 250 nursing clinics in operation today. They range from the makeshift, basement-of-the-local-church type where they check blood pressures, do elementary screening, and dispense simple advice to modern, free-standing, state-of-the-art, advanced practice meccas. But they all have one thing in common. *Not one is operating in black ink.*

Staff consists of nursing faculty and students who "volunteer" their time. To stay afloat they have to rely "on the kindness of strangers." They constantly petition (one said pester) corporations, institutions, and individuals for equipment, supplies, services, and cold, hard cash.

As one faculty member, who asked to remain anonymous, told me, "We're not teaching our students how to survive in the business world, we're teaching them the fine art of begging."

Nurses are always moaning, "But who is going to take care of the poor?" Why don't we ever moan, "But who is going to take care of the rich?"

I met a man who asked himself just that. He opened a home health agency that caters to the well-insured and well-endowed. One client demands round-the-clock registered nurses for which she pays him $100,000 a year. The client doesn't *need* professional nursing care, but when you have $20 million in the bank, you can have whatever you want.

The do-gooder in me just had to ask him about the poor people who couldn't afford such a service. He assured me he was sympathetic, but first and foremost he was a businessman. If he couldn't turn a profit, he couldn't stay in business long enough to take care of anyone.

Rose Memorial Hospital in Denver is just one hospital among many that provides upscale services for patients who are willing to pay. They have six private suites. For an additional $200 a day you can stay in one of the suites. They are beautifully furnished with original artwork on the walls, recessed lighting, and elegant bathrooms. Don't like what's on the menu? There is a chef on duty that will whip up whatever you want to eat.

John Bedrosian, executive vice president of the eminently profitable National Medical Enterprises, Inc., a company that owns or operates over 200 hospitals and long-term care facilities, says hospitals that fail to make a profit are mismanaged. They usually lack adequate inventory control, are not properly reimbursed by Medicare and Medicaid, and have poor controls on staffing. "You cannot have the luxury of too much nursing," he says.

". . . The luxury of too much nursing"—that phrase nearly leaped off the paper at me. Nursing as a luxury. I had thought of nursing as a need, a necessity, a right, a responsibility but never a *luxury*.

Could it be that we have missed our best bet: marketing professional nursing care as a luxury. Picture a commercial with a satisfied patient saying, "Sure, professional nursing care costs a little more, but *I'm* worth it."

Let's mount an offensive. Let's not wait for clients to come to us. Let's go for it! After all, "We're the most expensive nurses in America . . . and darn well worth it!"

Learn to Negotiate

The mark of a successful negotiation is that everyone leaves with some, if not all, of their needs satisfied. Nurses are just beginning to learn that almost everything in life is negotiable.

Here is a nurse who had a perfect opportunity to negotiate but muffed it:

> I was in the nursing office last week when our staffing coordinator was discussing a staffing dilemma with another nurse. I volunteered to work an extra night to help her out.

> What I should have negotiated was the fact that I really wanted Saturday night off. I should have said, "I will work the extra night *if* I can have Saturday night off." Needless to say, I worked Saturday and Sunday and have the extra night to "look forward to."

In this situation both the coordinator and the staff nurse have needs. The staff nurse volunteers to meet the coordinator's need without even expressing her own need. Now she is kicking herself. She had everything to gain and nothing to lose by negotiating.

If she had made the offer and the coordinator saw it as a satisfactory solution, both would have been happy. If the proposed solution solved one problem but created another, namely a Saturday shortage, it may not have worked. Since the proposal was contingent on a mutual satisfaction of needs, the staff nurse can gracefully withdraw saying, "It was just a suggestion. I'm sorry we couldn't work something out."

Nurses are so used to meeting others' needs while ignoring

their own that they lack experience in negotiating. Supervisors, used to having nurses volunteer with no strings attached, may be surprised as nurses gain some sophistication in negotiating skills.

Negotiations can range from getting one night off to collective bargaining for the whole institution. When negotiations break down, the ultimate solution is a strike. Many think a strike would be more correctly called the ultimate problem.

Strike! Few nurses are comfortable with that solution . . . or problem.

For years we have labored under the delusion that a nurses' strike would leave patients dying in the streets. But do you know what happens when doctors go on strike? The mortality *drops!* The most plausible explanation is that elective surgery is postponed and patients are sent home. (We all know a hospital is the worst place to be if you're sick.)

In actuality, a nationwide nurses' strike might save thousands of lives. Patients are in more jeopardy when nurses passively continue to work in spite of broken equipment, inadequate supplies, inept doctors, and a staff that is tired, ill-prepared, or inexperienced.

Make Sure the Solution Matches the Problem

Remember, implementing a solution is not the last step in the problem-solving process. Before you can lay the problem to rest, you have to evaluate the outcome. That evaluation determines whether a problem is truly solved or whether it needs to be reworked.

Nursing has an abundance of problems: unwieldy work loads, compressed salaries, inconsistent educational policies, subordinate status, subservient mentality, little respect, lack of autonomy, responsibility without authority, and limited opportunities for advancement—real or otherwise.

Perfectly good solutions for one problem are totally worthless when applied to other problems. Take advanced education. Although it may be a solution for some of the above problems, it is not a solution for all of those problems.

At a national meeting one irate nurse demanded to know just when her education was going to pay off. She had felt pressured to acquire her bachelor's and master's and was now working on her doctorate. Along the way she felt she had been promised that the solution to nursing's economic problems could be found in education. That promise was proving false, and she was mad as a hornet.

If you think education will improve your financial status, think again. At every point in the life cycle a male high school graduate will make more than a college-educated female. For 20 years the difference in average educational attainment between men and women has only been one tenth of a year. Men earn much more than women because they invest in a different type of educational capital. Women still invest in fine arts, teaching, nursing, and other social and service-oriented fields.

Upon completing a PhD, one nurse found herself more than $10,000 in debt. For her sacrifice and accomplishment, she received a $500 a year raise. With luck she thought she might recoup her investment before she retires.

If she had counted on advanced education to solve her financial problems, she would be as angry as the other nurse. Although the piddling monetary gain disappointed her, she found that her education would "pay off" in other ways. She was enjoying her new status, increased autonomy, unsolicited job offers, and opportunities for recognition in her specialty area. Education solved some of her problems, and, happily, they were the problems she found most pressing.

Expect Success

Our actions and our beliefs are inextricably intertwined. It's not the truth per se but what we *believe* to be true that guides our behavior. If we expect success, we will move steadily toward it. If we expect failure, we will move steadily toward that.

What you believe to be true about yourself is vitally important because every moment you move toward making your self-image a reality. Do you see yourself as marginal or magnificent? Intelligent? Decisive? Energetic? Creative? Successful? Respected? Professional?

Whether the adjectives you use to describe yourself are positive or negative, your actions will be directed toward making them accurate. That makes it wise to accentuate the positive and eliminate the negative.

The same holds true for the nursing profession. Our profession is also moving steadily toward making its collective self-image a reality. Is the image of nursing marginal or magnificent?

If you alter your beliefs about yourself or nursing, a change in behavior will occur. You can actually trick yourself into changing for better, for worse, for richer, for poorer, toward sickness, or toward health.

Behaviorists, of course, contend it is much easier to alter behavior than beliefs. They contend acting differently will bring about a compatible change in beliefs.

For example, if you want to appear confident, walk 25% faster. People will think that you are a person who really knows where she is going. As you walk along at a faster clip, you will actually begin to feel more confident. Soon you are a person who really knows where she is going.

To *survive,* you have to call a halt to self-defeating beliefs and behaviors. To *thrive,* you have to replace them with positive thoughts and actions.

STOP	START
Putting yourself in jeopardy—physically, mentally, emotionally, financially	Taking care of yourself—physically, mentally, emotionally, financially
Trying to rescue *everyone* (especially those who do not wish to be rescued)	Helping others accept responsibility for their own actions and problems
Dreaming	Planning
Wishing for good things	Working toward goals
Apologizing for what you are not	Rejoicing in everything you are
Conforming	Creating
Wishing others were more thoughtful or helpful	Asking for what you want and need
Trying to be *Supernurse*	Delegating
Fretting	Enjoying
Being defensive	Taking the offensive
Wasting your time, talent, and energy	Investing your time, talent, and energy
Taking orders	Taking command
Agonizing over how things *should* be	Making the best use of the world "as is"
Believing in magic	Believing in yourself

More than leaders, nursing needs cheerleaders. Nursing needs positively focused professionals who dare to raise their sights far beyond the survival threshold. Nursing needs professionals who want to thrive.

Pro-Nurse "Do-It-Yourself" Epilogue

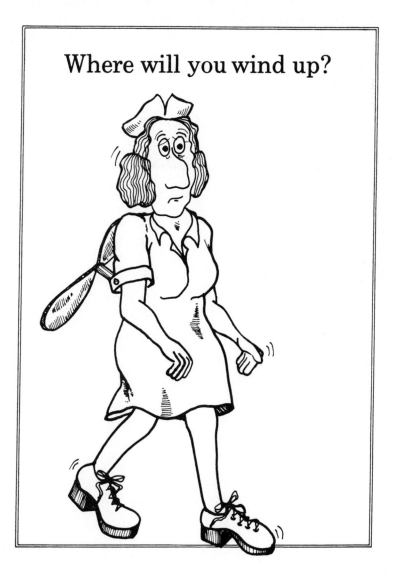

Where will you wind up?

ALL wound up and no place to go? Wishing that someone would point you in the right direction so you'd be all set?

Well, I can wind you up, but no one can point you in *the* right direction. There are all sorts of right directions. You have all the pain and pleasure of choosing your own.

Picking the right direction is only possible when you know where you want to go. It might help to think of your life as a short story and take Edgar Allan Poe's approach. He wrote the endings first. Then he worked backward so they came out as he desired.

Write your ending first. Make it grand. If you keep the end in sight, making decisions along the way is much less complicated. Remember, the heights you reach will depend more on your courage than your ability.

Where will you wind up?

It's your choice. Dare to make it.

INDEX